T0197190

THE SECOND
MESSAGE
ON MY
FOREARM

LYLE DE LEON

BALBOA.
PRESS

A DIVISION OF HAY HOUSE

Balboa Press books may be ordered through booksellers or by contacting:

Balboa Press
A Division of Hay House
1663 Liberty Drive
Bloomington, IN 47403
www.balboapress.com.au
1 (877) 407-4847

Because of the dynamic nature of the Internet, any web addresses or links contained in this book may have changed since publication and may no longer be valid. The views expressed in this work are solely those of the author and do not necessarily reflect the views of the publisher, and the publisher hereby disclaims any responsibility for them.

The author of this book does not dispense medical advice or prescribe the use of any technique as a form of treatment for physical, emotional, or medical problems without the advice of a physician, either directly or indirectly. The intent of the author is only to offer information of a general nature to help you in your quest for emotional and spiritual well-being. In the event you use any of the information in this book for yourself, which is your constitutional right, the author and the publisher assume no responsibility for your actions.

Any people depicted in stock imagery provided by Thinkstock are models, and such images are being used for illustrative purposes only. Certain stock imagery © Thinkstock.

Print information available on the last page.

ISBN: 978-1-5043-0128-2 (sc)
ISBN: 978-1-5043-0129-9 (e)

Balboa Press rev. date: 02/09/2016

CONTENTS

INTRODUCTION

I believe that there are some cloud of doubts that blur one's mind ...whether my experiences were fictional or not. I can assure you they were all TRUE!

You must have known that man has dual nature, the inner and the outer selves. This can be segmented into the earthly or the material and the spiritual. It can also be called the lower body and the higher body--the latter is that which has been neglected for countless generations.

Today, our earthly civilizations are increasingly wicked and adulterous compared to the past, according to Jesus to his disciples 2000 years ago. This is found in the Book of Matthew.

Jesus dictated (and other Ascended Masters) recently the last few years the messages through the chosen messenger, Tatyana Mickushina.

(http://www.theascendedmasters.com./index.html)

The recent dictations by the Ascended Hosts started in 2005 up to 2014.

There are a lot of worldly distractions which pull humanity towards the center of an infinite abyss, like a tornado, churning the lives and properties, devastating everything that it passes by.

Are we aware that our lives are like this? Similar to a powerful twister, our soul is pulled away from the real path...the Rose Path which the angels have given direction to the incarnating soul before he enters the human flexh. It seems to be forgotten once the soul is in the flesh.

The senses become attached to the physical world as one approaches adulthood. (But remember we have our past lives and had accumulated karma, negative or positive). The senses of the young gets slowly polluted as it parts from the teenage stage. He is exposed to many temptations that enhance pleasurable and sweet experiences. He is naturally taken, as he forgets the other world which sent him here to advance his soul.

We are told that the other world which cannot be seen in our world is more than a thousand times more beautiful than the world we are living in today.

We hardly believe this because we do not have the senses to see and feel the supernatural world. This is the main reason why the Ascended Masters have come to remind us about the end of this generation. (One zodiacal generation of souls is 12,000 years) is almost here.

In every flesh, the soul resides at the base of the brain (sella tursica). The New Testament tells us "that we are Gods" because at the core of the soul is a dazzling particle coming from God. The soul dictates the carnal mind the way to his Paternal Home. He is toned down or he does not seem to hear the silent reminders from the inner soul by the strong dominance of the earthly ego in man.

The harbor in the mind of man has been given the choice what to follow. But what has man done in the last 12,000 years? He followed the dictates of his carnal mind, making this world more dense, karmically. The field of negative Karma in which man has very meager knowledge. This Source has left no significance in his life in all his physical embodiments through the centuries because he has been misled by elders for their own gain.

Vices, such us gambling, watching indecent TV shows and CDs, indulging with harmful dangerous drugs and alcohol are just few examples. Yielding or entertaining thoughts of beautiful women and handsome men adds to the weight of negative karma which has accumatlated in time. Only a a handful in the evolving population has overcome worldly temptations,

These are they prophets and saints.

I have been told that I was an old soul. Many promptings were shown to me year after year as I was experiencing through the last 55 years. You will find these mystical experences in this little book.

I had been a victim of worldly attractions in my younger days and I have asked forgiveness from God for all the wickedness, and carelessness I did. I have been totally conscious of my sinful acts committed and today, I am poor but happy and I can claim I am a different man.

Since January 2012, after my by-pass operation two angels helped me (two weeks after the post-operative complications) which were unknown to the hospital staff. I have totally changed. The 31-day confinement was truly an incredibly disheartening experience! This has ultimately led me to the Inner Path.

I

THE TIME IS RIPE!

I was born on the 19th of September 1937, the first son of ten children.

Although I may have been trained scientifically in the medical profession, I profess I have neither proficiency nor intellectual distinction. As to how I became a physician makes a fascinating story. I never thought I would become a Doctor of Medicine. I was far below the average during my primary and elementary grades as well as in my first two years in high school. At age 16, my third year in 1953, I started to pick up a jot in my studies, so I graduated in my senior year as "first honorable mention," the third in a class of 42 members. In medical school, I was an average student. I assumed there was nothing exceptional about me but I was the president of our medical class from first year to the fourth year.

The world of the unknown or the fields of paranormal sciences are most often viewed with contempt, disdain or ridicule by some learned men, physical scientists and religious leaders who seemed to have lost their open-mindedness. Discussing matters of this kind is repugnant to some. Nevertheless, this is the field that stirs my imagination and interest.

My experiences somehow were strange. Extra-ordinary incidents made me accept there is a lot more to be learned from the metaphysical world beyond our limited scientific investigations.

A lot of books on these mysteries have been written for centuries. But only a small portion of the population is interested in reading them. The truth of the matter is that the scientific sphere takes little cognizance of such mysteries. Some fields have gained little acceptance by some physical scientists. Some scientists investigate the galaxies and the Universe to prove that there is no God. The Hubble telescope exhibited wonderful and beautiful images of the galaxies and made some scientists more confused but some held to their belief in a Maker.

There were many unique and strange encounters I experienced which made me lean towards the study of intuitive feelings as well as the psychic phenomena that relate to the mystifying world of the unknown. Were some extraterrestrial beings behind these mystical encounters?

I was in a quandary in my early years over the paranormal happenings in my life and some people's lives. Rather than ignore them as skeptics do, I regarded them significant. These lured me as unnatural, rather than normal, attractions.

In l961, I was a freshman medical student when I had my future read when I wandered in the streets of Manila one weekend. This "Fortune Teller" had a crystal ball and told me of my future events, and at one point, she said 'You will be going abroad.' I never thought of going abroad. Going abroad I did, when I was 41 in l976. It took that long to happen (15 years). I was able to secure a Visa only for 30 days but stayed on for as I had become an Australian citizen.

After six months, the Medical Superintendent asked me if I wished to stay in Australia. I had been an illegal migrant then. The superintendent must have liked my performance, as he immediately worked for my permanent residency.

After a few years, I began to be interested in paranormal activities, and met some mediums or clairvoyants.

Mediums or clairvoyants have been scorned or loathed in the Christian world for centuries. This was true with the prophets of old. Why? This is due to the biblical injunction that did not allow contact with the dead. The biblical taciturnity that contact with the dead was prohibited.

It was King Saul, the enemy of David, who wanted David, killed because of his extreme jealousy: he had been told by a medium that one day the throne would be handed to David. This prediction was made after David killed Goliath. To block the ascension of David to the throne, King Saul banned all mediums. It was King Saul, the enemy of David, who wanted David killed because of his extreme jealousy: The fact that one day the throne would be handed to David according to a medium. This evolved after David killed Goliath. To block this, King Saul banned all the mediums. Nobody was allowed to contact the dead for guidance or predictions of future events. **Yet, at his last cling to life, King Saul consulted a medium, the witch of Ensor, and Samuel identified himself and talked to King Saul of his impending doom. Samuel said if the king changed his attitude, his life would be spared.**

King Saul could have saved his life had he stopped his serious intent to get rid of David. He could have given up the throne without much bloodshed. It was King Saul's pride and jealousy that led to his own destruction together with his beloved son. Not because he consulted a medium as some claim as the cause of King Saul's and son's demise. The main reason was that he did not follow the instruction that was given by Samuel.

There are numerous incidents written in the Old and New Testaments that deal with the paranormal. The Holy Bible, after all, is concerned with the spiritual progress of man.

Almost three quarters of the book deal with prophecy. To the agnostics, the metaphysical level does not exist.

In Nature everything is an exchange of energy, either physical and tangible or intangible. The physical Universe is 4.6 % tangible energy. The rest is dark matter and dark energy. It is not because we cannot see the cosmic waves and dark energy. There are things we do not see like radio waves, telephony, electricity or television signals. But cosmic waves are a great source of energy as are astral projections, the 6th sense, premonitions, insights and dark energy. No matter how they are called, these forces exist. Animals are born with a sixth sense. We have lost some of this sixth sense as humans evolved in the last few million of years.

The work of professionals especially in the field of astrology is to learn to control the interpretation of these energies over years of hard work and experience. We are all born with different innate capacities and some are more sensitive than others to these forces.

A great number of people today have been indoctrinated by their religious beliefs. They have become prisoners of their own creed or religious doctrines. There is no allowance for broad-mindedness, only restraints. Open-mindedness has been controlled by their superiors.

It was told 2000 years ago: 'Seek and ye shall find; knock and it shall be opened unto you!' To me, these words meant knocking at the door of the spiritual realm—the metaphysical world. Paranormal states like intuition, extra-sensory perception (ESP), clairvoyance, astral projections, the superconscious state and other related fields are difficult for the scientific world to investigate. To these unbelievers, the world is plainly physical in its dimensions, but believers are able to perceive dimensions of energy that are unseen by the human eyes, yet are alive, active and vibrating on their own all over the Universe. After all only 4.6 per cent of the physical universe can be seen and felt. The rest are unseen. Yet there are millions of threads that other creations use to allow them to travel to every corner of the countless galaxies.

In my view, the metaphysical state made this world exist but with supernatural boundaries. A select number of individuals are given this knowledge. They act as windows to the ethereal realm. Clairvoyants appreciate and feel its existence through this window. They are "gifted," sometimes solving a murder which detectives can't solve. The mystical world has complete control of the physical world without our conscious knowledge. Man is totally left to his own free will to knock and search into this metaphysical state.

Use of Free Will is a birthright for all. It is sad to see how some cultures have taken away the rights of individuals. Knocking on this door may not be given or answered. Submission to the Will of his Creator does not necessarily mean the answer will be available. It is through the "gifted individuals that information may be given" partly or fully. Even God does not know what the Will of man decides.

A very thin segment of human society is given the ability or gift to comprehend the Supernatural level. But everybody is gifted with intuition which comes in varying degrees. Yet most people do not feel they have it.

There are other gifts that provide a certain dimension when occasions call for it. For instance, laying of hands for healing has been known for ages. Others may demonstrate clairvoyance. Some may have it although clouded or limited, but to some gifted individuals, clairvoyance produces exquisite results.

The gift of prophecy has been demonstrated by many in history. Did John the Apostle show it? Or the famous Nostradamus? Or the Mayan prophets or the ancient Egyptian prophets as written in stone walls? All these manifestations emerge in varying degrees of clarity. Nevertheless, not one of the psychic phenomena manifested among these rare individuals can show a deep and distinct depth of mysticism. There was always a demarcation line.

A tinge of cloudiness may blur the full significance of an event. Even in the case of the foremost American Sleeping Prophet, Edgar Cayce, a few things were not revealed, 'These are not to be revealed,' said Edgar Cayce when asked during a "reading" while in a trance. Varying forms of mysticism have appeared throughout history and in every culture.

I worked for nine years in the hinterlands in the Philippines where the culture was very primitive. There was one elderly who could tell that death was impending when a person passed by the front of his house (without his knowledge). He could see some kind of aura. He could predict the death of that individual in a few days. This was hard to believe. As far as I know, this kind of paranormal occurrence never happened in cities.

There is an extreme restriction of this knowledge. In most cases, this knowledge is given out partially. This is the reason why some predictions by mediums come true, some partially. In earlier times mediums were accused of sorcery. In medieval times, their head or neck would be cut off, or they would be burned at the stake. It is written in the Old Book: 'To some knowledge is given full, to some little, to some none at all.'

Some of us have had unusual or mysterious experiences in our lives. Some have had strong intuition and strange encounters. I am certain most have had experiences that almost claimed their lives or limbs. One can only say, 'Boy was I lucky!' 'It was a miracle, I survived a plane crash.' Given enough time to review his life and dig deep into the unusual happening -- he or she will discover that we truly live in a mysterious world. Sometimes I wonder why I have had so many mystical experiences.

These experiences mystify me. There seemed to be an entity or entities present as if someone was snatching me from the tentacles of death or an impending catastrophe.

I have wondered the last 60 years regarding these mysterious incidents, insignificant though they may have been at their time of occurrence. All that is written here are my true experiences. I leave these mysteries to your understanding.

These encounters have become a portion of my life, a life that I consider fulfilling, puzzling in its course, mystical it may seem in its roots, but forming a whole reality that is coming now to its end.

Spiritual and earthly evolution had to take place. What I could not discern was the statement of the American Sleeping Prophet, Edgar Cayce, that the past, present, and future are one. To me, the present as we experience today, happened already a long time ago. Are we in an infinite cycle? We are not there yet. We are assured by Inelia Benz, sent by the Source; that we will be there in a few generations. Our technological advancement has been hidden from us by the greed of the wealthy bloodlines or the elite group.

When we evolve into higher dimensions, we can travel in time and space. This will come in the future.

Time and space exist as one. Not as we understand time and space in our planet. When we are there, we can travel following the millions of threads out there in the Universe. We can go back and forth, from the past to the future. Is it not a better place to live in, at no expense?

My spiritual understanding of this world was changed slowly during the last few years. Today is the 15th of March 2013. After reading a lot of the exposes and disclosures of a few individuals in their retirement years who had contacts with aliens for many years, some in their early childhood like Bob Dean, Dr. Steve Greer, and the incarnation of Inelia Benz, I began to have good thoughts as regards the "spirits" who had guided me throughout my life, though unseen.

Please open the websites of Project Camelot, Project Avalon, Exopolitics, Jordan Maxwell, Laura Eisenhower, Inelia Benz, Intellihub.com, White Hats.com and many others that you can search in the Internet. You will have a better understanding of what is happening in the world today, knowledge which has been kept hidden from the public for decades by the elite. Who are they?

About a week before my 75th birthday while still asleep at about 5:00 in the morning somebody grabbed my hair and shook my head once. After an hour I decided to get up. I asked my wife (there were only two of us in the house) why she grabbed my hair and shook my head. She never woke me up like this before. She denied doing either. I thought then that I just had a dream. It seemed so real.

A few days later, at about the same time, somebody grabbed my right leg, flexed it 90 degrees, and pulled my leg. I asked my wife why she did those things, but she again denied doing any of it. Then I began to think that it must be the "spirit" that has been protecting me throughout my life. It was suggesting that I use my head and go on with what I was supposed to do. It was time to continue writing the fact that I was not trained as a writer or journalist.

The day I opened my computer, without my searching for it, Project Camelot came on the screen. Later that day, I realized I was being led to this site. It was my first time to be exposed to this website. The next few weeks I was engrossed by the disclosures and histories of some individuals who had long contacts with extra-terrestrial beings. (You can find this in the Archives of Project Camelot.) Some of them had been invited to other planets in our galaxy. Did the voice that talked to me when I was 19 years old, the possession by a spirit when I was 30, the appearance of Jesus Christ in the cloud when I was 48, and a lot more, were these done by malevolent extraterrestrial beings? The two humanoid "angels" that helped saved my life too? (They appeared when I had a complicated open heart surgery in January 2011.) Was the "spirit guide" that grabbed my hair and pulled my leg recently the same guide that had watched over me throughout my life? I can say now 'Yes, he must be the same guide.'

The clairvoyant I knew very well told me (in 1985) that I had two guides -- the archangel Michael, and a "Holy Ghost." I asked her who the 'Holy Ghost' was. She answered "Elijah." I only know of one Elijah--the Prophet. Was Elijah from the highest ultra-dimension or from the Source? Most of us know that Elijah was from God.

According to Bob Dean, there are 200 civilizations in our galaxy and 57 have visited the earth. There are 400 billion stars in our galaxy and 400 billion galaxies in our Universe. We are then one of the tiniest creations in our galaxy. Edgar Cayce mentioned universes beside our own. This reduces our planet to a quantum particle. According to unique genius David Wynn Miller there are ETs who are still present in Greenland under the ice structures that are 85 feet tall. Is this hard to believe!

Who created us? According to those who have befriended the ETs, we have been genetically created at least 50,000 years ago. That is more recent compared to extraterrestrial aliens whose civilizations are thousands and even a million years ahead of us. We are lagging far behind in our quest for advancement! Half of our genes belong to the outside world. Would you believe they come from the Annunaki?

Why? Because we have been stunted in our spiritual growth by greed and wars among ourselves in our planet. The benevolent ETs are trying to prevent the Third World War which will be nuclear. Will we have nuclear devastation? The ETs started to come to help us when the atomic bombs were dropped in Japan. There have been many UFO sightings in the UK and USA (especially in Arizona) after World War II.

Why are the extraterrestrials interested in us? Is it because we are beautiful people in this planet? We have seen faces of aliens whose photos were taken (their craft had landed or crashed accidentally) in Africa or New Mexico or nearby states. They don't look handsome or pretty. Most of the inhabitants of this earth will be scared if the ETs materialize themselves physically.

The spirituality of humanity will save us if we can remove the walls that divide the races of man. The ETs can detect and read our thoughts and behavior with their advance science. They have sent "modern prophets" to Earth like Inelia Benz and a few others to raise individual vibrations into oneness, or collectiveness as a whole. Are we heeding the silent call?

The human flesh was genetically created by scientific beings from other planets but not our souls. Our souls had existed for eons, and had been created by the Supreme Creator. This time, our wandering souls are allowed to incarnate or use the human flesh on this planet for its advancement.

The flesh and its brain that had been genetically molded by the aliens have not followed the path that our creators (scientists from other planets) created for us. Are there aliens that are benevolent among malevolent ones (the Reptilians, Arcons, Grays) in our setting? Did the ET design greed and selfishness in our genes? Which one is to blame? Is it the human flesh or the malevolent aliens? The soul registers the thoughts and the deeds of the flesh and all are recorded in another planet known as Akasia (according to Edgar Cayce). This vehicle, this body, whatever it does—has been held captive by the indwelling soul and is freed only when the body is physically dead. Through its existence this has been recorded in the soul's mind, all thoughts and acts, and a duplicate in the book of Remembrance or the Akashic record.

I now believe that my guides after all these decades were the good extraterrestrial beings.

The Reptilians are the bad ETs! These bad apples are hiding and the good ETs are after them.

Some reptilian ETs have incarnated in the flesh of the wealthy on this planet; some are disguised as earthly beings. They have the control of the elite and the elitist are hiding truths from the public. Why hide them? So they can control the economy of many countries by controlling oil and oil products for their own benefit. There were discoveries in the early part of the century but they have covered them to prevent the advancement of our science. We should be travelling from city to city or from planet to distant stars with electromagnetic force by now. Lift tons of rocks with our fingers with an anti-gravity gadget. But they have succeeded to hide this knowledge. We should be able to de-materialize ourselves as the ETs do. This is the main reason why a few retired heroes from the military have come out to disclose the truth. Others have been murdered or had met "accidents" because they started to leak out information or did not want to cooperate. Whose decision was the evil act? Is it the ETs? Or is it the consciousness of the top guys and the elite? These bad apples are so difficult to find. They can make themselves appear and disappear!

The disclosures of these individuals are slowly leaking into the public. Not everybody who comes to this knowledge is enlightened. In due time, many will be convinced. As for me, I believe this is my mission in life: To help reveal the hidden truth and awaken the masses to what is going to happen.

If some who had disclosed information had disappeared or had accidents or were murdered, then we can conclude that those responsible for their disappearance or death are indeed evil. One individual reported that he could not stay more than an hour in the underground base in Arizona because "they" were mutilating human bodies. What for? Who were the dissectors? Were they extraterrestrial aliens? But they know the science of our bodies as part and parcel of our physical creation. Why mutilate? Or are there aliens from another galaxy who don't know our earthly physical beings? Or are they earthly human dissectors? This must be, for they have an insatiable appetite just as the Romans loved to see blood when Christians were mutilated and devoured in the arena by lions.

Aliens and the greedy folks have built during the last 60 years luxurious underground bases in many countries using the people's tax money. Their reason: it is the task of the military and chosen intellectuals to keep the existence of such bases a secret so people will not panic. Is it? Will the time be late? When the time comes a lot of people will be dying from hunger and disease. Or is it their design? It was so designed so they can establish the New World Order! And who were responsible for the creation of the Georgia Guidestones? Nobody could trace them but they were fully paid to build the structure. Were they ordered by malevolent aliens?

The New World Order will be governed by greedy folks where no religions will flourish and the rest will just be slaves. Will this ever happen? It is prophesied that the new World Order will be a peaceful Social Order. Where there will be no wars anymore. What will happen to those who are hiding in underground bases? Have they created their own tombs?

The road will be bumpier in the next decade. A lot of lives will be lost. Just hold on tight!

II

MY TRUE LIFE EXPERIENCES

I will write down my metaphysicial experiences throughout my life as printed in the first book. I hope this will reach more folks around the globe. Whether you believe my unusual experiences, it is for you to believe or refuse to believe.

What do you intend to do? Are you not interested to go into the real world? Are you not not going to prepare your mind? Please act now!

1

MY MOTHER'S SECRET

Whenever my mother was asked to give a message in church decades after World War II, she related that her near-death-experience (NDE) then coming back to life was a miracle... Although she did not have any training in homiletics, she did very well when she delivered her sermons.

The NDE experience made her a devout follower of Jesus Christ. She fostered spiritual fulfillment in herself especially when she became the national president of the Women's Association of the Philippines in the 1960s. In her dream during her NDE. She told me about this dream when I was already 49 years old.

The places where the family evacuated during World War II were 20 kilometers or more from one another. When the war broke out, my father was the certified public accountant of a lumber company in Anakan, a barrio in the town of Gingoog, Misamis Oriental in the north-eastern part of the island of Mindanao. The American manager of the company requested the Philippine Recruitment Authority not to order my father to join the army because he was badly needed to operate the company. My father was exempted from the draft, and the lumber mill continued to operate, but not for long. Japanese soldiers invaded the camp, and when reports of their cruelty became rampant, the employees fled to the mountains, some, including our family, to barrios distant from the town. The lumber mill stopped operation.

My family and a few close friends formed a group and lived in one place. The families stayed there for a few months; they cleared small patches of light forest areas and planted them with root crops, bananas, and fast-growing crops. One day someone brought the message that a Japanese patrol was a few kilometers away. The families packed their belongings in a hurry, leaving behind their growing crops.

From the shorelines, the Japanese soldiers were merciless. They would go deeper into areas accessible by road. Our families had to contend with two enemies – the invading soldiers, and, from the jungles, the Bagobo natives. Families were caught between the two warring forces. The Bagobos, known to be head hunters, attacked at night, looted, and killed children, women, and men while they were sleeping in their native *cogon* (a species of monocot grass) or nipa huts.

My parents and a few family friends banded together and managed to escape from the two forces by travelling at dusk to dawn. The little kids were carried on the shoulders of the men who had not been called to join the Philippine Army.

Hiding in secluded places, the evacuees had to deal with the Anopheles mosquito, carrier of the malaria parasite. The deadly killer claimed the lives of some evacuees. There were no pharmaceutical drugs to treat people with malaria. People pinned their hopes on the native medicine coming from the bark of a tree known as "dita" or cinchona, from which the Atabrine tablet was developed. The bark was boiled, and the bitter liquid was taken by mouth. Three cups of the concoction had to be taken daily when one was suspected of coming down with malaria.

A number of families were unfortunate. If the Japanese did not find them, the head hunters raided them at night, looted their belongings and burned their temporary shelters. Those caught were speared or hacked to death. If they did not die from the rifles of the Japanese or the spears of the primitive tribes, malaria would strike them down if they could not get hold of the bark of the cinchona tree. A few families escaped those two enemies. My family was one of them. Did we have a guardian angel watching over us?

I can still recall being carried on the shoulder of a man as we crossed rivers and hills for two days to find a safer place the Japanese could not reach. We passed through the interiors of the province of Misamis Oriental and the adjoining province of Agusan. It was not safe to pass through dilapidated roads. The Japanese patrols where everywhere. The safest way was to follow rugged trails then head for the seashore where friends guided us to a small village by the seaside known as Binuagan, now a large town. There were only number families in the village at that time.

The barely noticeable village was hidden from the road. A cluster of diptherocarp rainforest trees surrounded the area. Contact was made with close friends. One of them was Rev. Pedro Raterta family. The head of the family would become a Bishop of the United Church of Christ in the Philippines two decades after the war.

At the new evacuation site, my mother was prey to the Anopheles mosquito. She had to be carried by hammock made of rattan vines which was suspended by a bamboo pole and carried by two adults. My father tried to help carry the hammock, but he was dissuaded from doing so as he had developed severe joint pains. My mother was seven months pregnant with her fifth child. This was delivered pre-maturely. Later she lost the baby boy from severe malnutrition.

Months later, we were able to establish a hideout in a hidden cove in Goso-on with a few families. A thick tropical forest by the seaside covered Goso-on, near Punta Diwata, in Misamis Oriental. Our hideout could not be seen by Japanese war planes or ships from the sea. We stayed in that safe place for almost two years until the surrender of Japan. I remember the leaflets scattered from American planes overhead, declaring, "War is over. Japan has surrendered."

Going back to October 1943, a year after the war broke out, my mother had severe malaria. Chills, high fever, headaches and loss of appetite gripped her. She could not eat anything solid for 28 days. She had to be forced to drink small amounts of water and broth so she will not dehydrate severely. Sometimes she was comatose. The liquid from the boiled bark of a cinchona tree that was very bitter was forced into her throat. (Atabrine tablets came later when the Americans liberated the Philippines.) She became severely dehydrated, very pale, and weak. Her legs could not support her body when she tried to get up. I believe she had contracted the severe form of malignant malaria

Her end seemed to be near when she was comatose for two days. "She would soon pass into the other world," family friends who had gathered around her early one evening said. Candido Tan, a devout and kind Christian, was sure she was going to die in a few minutes. He related later when she seemed to get her last breath, the words uttered by my mother as she was slowly fading away, her breathing shallow, her face and skin ashen gray, and her pulse could hardly be felt.

The paragraphs below are excerpts from the book my mother wrote, *My Pilgrimage of Faith* in the 1980s. Despite her frail health during the war, she could recall vividly her experience of having died and reaching heaven. She was not dreaming, she said. If it was an ordinary dream, she would have forgotten about it in a day or two. But she never forgot it, and remembered every detail of her experience until she died at age 79. She wrote:

It was as though I had been walking a very long way and came upon a wide plain. The scenery was beautiful! I had not seen such beauty in my whole life. The air was cool and soothing to the skin and was sweetened by the perfume of beautiful flowers that stretched as far as the eyes could see. Their colors rippled in the sunlight – red and pink, gold and white. Butterflies danced over them, performing the dance of Nature. Amidst that sea of beauty

I exclaimed: "Oh how beautiful! What a beautiful country!" I walked and walked and wandered wherever my feet took me, enjoying cool perfumed air, the sunshine and the flowers. Then I came upon stumps of wood placed in graduated heights to form a stairway. I climbed this ladder of stumps and once on top I beheld a sight far more beautiful than the one below the stairs. The flowers were more abundant and larger. From where I stood, I could see a road made of gold. I walked down this road, then slid down like a little child, and kissed the flowers on the roadside now and then. No such beauty, indeed, had I seen in my life before. I was alone yet I was not lonely. There was not a memory of where I came from, of my former existence. Everything was so serene, nothing seemed to make me ruffled or excited. I was just happy!

Soon I realized that the road of gold led to a place enclosed by high walls of glittering multi-colored stones. Standing by the gate, I saw from above the walls that it was brightly lighted inside as if some great show was going on. There was an old pot-bellied man by the gate with long gray hair and beard, looking like Santa Claus. He slept and snored loudly. I tried to awaken him to announce my arrival but he rolled his head to the other side and snored even more loudly. I ran down the road again, kissed the flowers and chased the butterflies, stopping every time I would feel pain in the area just below my navel. I sat on the road, pressing my belly, and said 'Ouch!' When the pain subsided I went back to the old man and tried to awaken him, but it was only at my fourth try that he opened his eyes. I told him, I had come and waited for a long time but he had been sound asleep and would not wake up.

"Oh, but I did not insist that you should come," the old man said, because you pleaded hard not to be asked to leave your husband and children because they are all sick.

"Then thank you so much, Sir if you send me home because my husband and children are sick and there is no one to take care of them except for a 12-year-old girl. She might be called away by her mother any time. Before I go, may I see God? I requested.

"Yes, but not the father,' the old man replied. He is too strong a light for your eyes. However, you can see Jesus."

All at once I saw Jesus walk from my left to the right, dressed in the long familiar garment with a top robe of red. He was carrying a little girl in his arm and holding another girl by the hand, the sizes of my two girls, Louella and Domini, aged four and three. As quickly as Jesus and the two girls appeared, they disappeared. I turned to the old man, thanked him, and said goodbye. I slid down the road.

I had not gone very far when I began to notice that where I stood, there sprouted human beings from the ground. I tried to touch them but felt nothing. I exclaimed, "Is this a graveyard? Surely this must be John 3:28. All of a sudden I felt a force that seemed to carry me towards a crowd and I struggled, crying, "No, please, I'm not going. I'm not dead yet." "Just come and you shall see," said a voice that sounded like that of the old man at the gate.

I could not do anything. I moved with the crowd as in a parade and we walked through a beautiful boulevard with tall trees on both sides. I could hear the rustle of footsteps but could not see anybody. As we walked past the trees I heard the old man say, "This is your place, 'This is yours,' and "You, the next one," and so on as if he was assigning places for everyone in the crowd. The sound of steps became fewer and fewer until I came to the last tree. And then I heard a voice addressing me, "Now you may go home, you have no place here yet." Then I woke up as if I had awakened from a deep sleep."

When everybody thought my mother was going to give up the ghost, she sat up, opened her eyes, moved her face around, and joined the people who were singing a hymn of mourning. They finished the hymn and everybody was more than surprised. She was alive! She asked who the man seated beside her was (my father). She could not recognize the people around her. My father wanted to comfort her and cuddle her but she pushed him away, saying loudly, "Go away, I am a married woman. My husband will kill you if he saw you with me!" She did not recognize him or her children -- except one. That was me! My mother recognized me! She called my name and hugged me.

I looked at the emaciated faces of the people who were there. They were all astonished at her sudden coming to life. **Was this a miracle?**

It was getting very dark and somebody lit the oil lamp and placed it on top of a small wooden box, a foot high from my mother's side near me. I felt the serenity of that fleeting moment. Solemn faces had gathered close around her. The small fragile faces of my two little sisters and tiny brother glittered faintly from the flickering light of the lamp. My vision started to become blurry. After a brief while, I could not recognize faces any more. Tears trickled down my cheeks, and a lump formed in my throat. Deep inside me had been deep sorrow; I thought Mama was going to die. And then, there she was, so alive and well.

I can still picture her convalescence vividly. She tried very hard to regain her strength and learn to walk again as she clung to a rope strung from one side of the room to the other. She strengthened her limbs slowly by walking back and forth inside our hut many times a day. My father could not do much as he was suffering from multiple joint pains.

Weeks passed, and my mother's frail slim legs finally supported her body weight without her clutching at the rope. She was on her way to recovery.

When my mother wrote the story in her book there was a portion she omitted. That was her recognizing me, and not her other children. I suppose, she did not want to hurt the feelings of the younger ones. But her siblings always thought I was her favorite child. When I went to college, Abigail the sixth child born after the war (the 4th child died during the evacuation period) became her pet. Somehow there was still a strong bond between my mother and me that was difficult to discern. In my growing years, I felt this closeness to my mother. I tried not to show this especially when my younger brothers and sisters were around. There were nine living kids in the family. I never did want to hurt Mama's feelings nor provoke her anger nor be disobedient except on the few occasions I acted like a stubborn boy. Of course, I felt bad for my pranks, but I tried to compensate silently by becoming more obedient.

When I went to college at age 17 and in the years that followed, my father always reminded me whenever he went for a side-trip to Silliman University, in Dumaguete City, where I took my pre-medical schooling, that I should write often to my mother. He said that she always missed me and shed tears very often, longing for me. At 23 years of age, when I was in proper medical school, my father came up to Manila once or twice a year. He would leave a note saying, "Your mother is often lonely for you and cries at night. Please write her often."

I was not a baby anymore, I told myself. I could not spend time writing her. I had nothing to write anyway. I had many things to do. She had the younger ones (eight of them) to keep her busy. Was I cruel to her? I neglected the plea. I was foolish and selfish and I never realized how this little gesture of writing was precious to her. Now I could feel how lonely one could be away from a loved one. Heartaches develop. When Mama died, I would feel empty and lonely, and tears would run down my cheeks in the middle of the night.

I wrote two or three times a year but very briefly. Oftentimes I just jotted a few words and sent a nearly blank page by mail. Of course, that was not enough, but it was enough for a mother to know that I was well. I guess some boys find it hard to write long letters unlike girls who can write pages for hours.

Growing up to maturity means a lot to most people. Parting with your parents may develop that attitude, "I don't want to be treated like a child!" A mother's feeling for her children will always be there, regardless of their age. That invisible navel seems to be connected even if time has changed the young mother to a graying elderly, and the young boy to a gentleman. I tried to escape subconsciously from getting extra attention since I left for college. Even after graduation from medical school, I went to practice my profession in a remote area of northern Luzon, in a mission hospital, more than 1000 miles away from home. I later realized how much my mother had wanted me to practice in Gingoog, our hometown, as she was proud of her son's being a medical doctor. In Mayoyao, where I busied myself treating the sick, I was still single but never felt alone. I felt I still did not want to arouse jealousy in my siblings especially after my father told me that Mama told her once, "How come it's only Nell that I miss so much?" Papa told me this story a year before he passed away in 1963.

Over the 28 years since my father died Mama endured loneliness. She kept herself busy at home, in local politics, in church work, in tending her flower garden and teaching dressmaking in her vocational school. She extended help to others and propagated the faith that she treasured so much. She began her morning reading the Bible and praying at a corner of the balcony in our two-story house in Cabuyoan subdivision.

One thought that my mother shared often was this: "Life itself is a pilgrimage, but much faith makes the hardest road easy and the heaviest load lighter." That was indeed very true. Her life was a struggle, with loads of burdens and tribulations but her profound faith made things comfortably bearable.

I migrated to Australia in 1976 and my family followed me after 12 months. I had four children, two boys and two girls. After 15 years out of sight from my mother, she was able to immigrate to Australia in 1983. She left many dear friends in the Philippines. She was with me the last eight years of her life.

She was contented with her retiring years. Then in 1985, she was diagnosed to have Multiple Myeloma, a form of cancer of the bone. She suffered a lot from this. Her back pains worsened the last two years, and she agonized in bed as she moved, and sometimes tears streamed down her cheeks.

She did not say any negative word against her Maker but continued to read the Bible which gave her comfort. She kept herself busy when she felt better. She did not prefer morphine or any strong analgesic. She still cooked, prepared a good menu, and sewed clothes for her grandchildren and friends whenever she could. She loved doing things for others. With the little things she could do with her hands, she made others happy and that happiness bounced back to her. Her kind acts were very appreciated by the recipients.

The last league of her journey at 77 seemed happy, and she looked contented though she may have been in agony. Analgesics relieved her pain at times. However, she was also missing the other children in the Philippines, especially the fifth in the family, Abigail, who was very talented but later suffered a nervous breakdown.

Mother wanted to do everything for her fifth child but she could only do so much. It was hurting her, the thought that her brightest child was gone. At times she asked God what she did wrong. This was the most painful thing she felt during the last ten years of her life. Many times I would say to her when she was in distress, "We should not challenge God by questioning Him but accept the things God has bestowed to us every day." I would add, "Is it not that everyday God has something set for us? It is for us to choose which is right to do."

She knew she was dying. Only time could tell. She wanted very much to see her old friends and the rest of the children back in the Philippines before her time came. A plane ticket was purchased. Everything was packed: gifts and personal belongings. She had the strong hope of returning to Australia after a planned three -month holiday in the country of her birth.

One night, a few days before departure, she started to bleed from her colon. She was in the hospital for four days. The doctors could not control the hemorrhage. Colonoscopies and gastroscopies were performed to locate the endless bleeding, and bottles of blood were pumped into her bloodstream. Finally, exploratory laparotomy showed she was bleeding continuously from the linings of her gut. On the third day, she developed DIC (Disseminated Intravascular Coagulation). The doctors tried everything. While in hospital, with all the procedures, repeated intravenous fluids, blood transfusions, she never uttered a single complaint. One doctor said she was a perfect patient, but they could only do so much for her.

Her eighth child, 36 at that time and I, 52, were by her side during the last two hours of her life. This was in the Intensive Care Unit of Blacktown District Hospital, New South Wales. We comforted her, read her passages from the Bible. She knew her time was nearing and submitted herself to God's will. When I kissed her checks for the last time, she kissed my cheeks too as if I was a baby. There was a warm and gentle sniff from her nostrils. She whispered: "Take care of your brothers and sisters." The words she spoke were hardly audible as her larynx had been irritated by the endotracheal tube.

She died on the 29th of April 1989. She was prepared to meet her Savoir.

Now I can tell you the secret she kept all the time regarding the dream that she did not write about in her book. Three years before she died, she told me that during World War II, when everyone believed she was at death's door, she was told to takes care of all the children, *"especially the eldest because God has a design for him."*

"God has a design for all," I reminded her.

"There may be something else behind those simple words," she added, "just be patient and wait."

I did not know then what God's design for me was.

Does God really have a design for me? What is it? At 48 years of age I started to feel the calling.

At 73 I understood and accepted my life's destiny.

At 75 my concept changed.

SURPRISED AT MYSELF!

I was 11 years old when this experience happened. I was in my 5th Grade in Masbate, a province in the Central Islands of the Visayas, Philippines. My father had established a lumber yard in this capital town. However, the business failed, and two years later we went back to Gingoog.

I was always a shy, timid and nervous boy. My heart fluttered, my knees trembled, and my voice quivered whenever I was called to recite in front of the class or at small gatherings. I dreaded singing a song or reciting a poem. In school, I refused sometimes to answer the teacher in long sentences even if I knew the answer. I would feel the tremors in my vocal chords. Words faltered, and my jaws would tighten up. I was a typical withdrawn pupil, ashamed and unsure of myself. I was utterly an introvert in the early stages of my early boyhood which I carried partly into adulthood.

One day, I was asked by my teacher to talk about the functions of the digestive system. For the first time I felt confident. There was no hesitation on my part, I went to the front of the class and discussed the subject matter expertly. Everyone listened. I was flawless for about 15 minutes.

To me, it was a surprise! The things I read the previous night were fresh in my mind. Usually, I could not retain the ideas I read. This time I did. The mind that I had was unbelievable! This must be the mind of the bright ones in the class. How I wished the "bright feeling" would stay on. I would be the valedictorian in our class, I thought if this continued. I would impress the very attractive light-skinned girl in my class (half bred – a mixture of Spanish and Filipino blood). Her eyes were so tantalizing that every boy in class was attracted to her.

My wish was not granted even in the years to come. Only the memory of it lingers.

3

THE FLYWHEEL

I was 13 when we moved back to a new home in Gingoog town, now a city. My mother opened a dress shop which later became a vocational school for dressmaking. My father, who was a certified public accountant by profession, opened a small printing press.

One day, I watched a printer form a mold out of types made of lead from the keyboards. He placed this on a steel frame on a table made of hard wood. He tightened the mold with a jigsaw arrangement of pieces of hard wood and quoins. Afterwards, the mold was clamped to the printing machine. The first printing machine we had resembled the Gutenberg type. We used foot power to keep it running. As soon as the flywheel gained its momentum, it was easy to run the press with one foot, then, when the foot became tired, change to the other foot. This was good exercise. It really made us sweat out especially on a hot summer day.

I taught myself everything in the printing press from type-setting to book-binding. Before long I was making diaries and selling them to my classmates so I could make a few pesos.

After a short while the printing business improved. We had more orders. Using foot power 14 hours a day was tiring, and production was limited. A year later, father bought a small 12-HP gasoline engine; this improved the business a bit. A 4-inch wide conveyor belt was attached to the flywheel and beeswax was applied to prevent the belt from slipping.

At times, the gasoline engine went haywire and revved up on its own. This made the flywheel turn very fast. The half-ton printing machine shook down to its foundation. The noise it created was so frightening I thought the whole engine would break into pieces. The two rollers made the most noise as if one was in a fast train running in a tunnel at full speed. Nobody could hand-feed the paper into the press as it flipped over a hundred impressions a minute or probably more. Whenever this engine ran very fast the printer-operator or whoever was closest to the engine would rush and adjust the carburettor wiring. This slowed down the machine. The noise it created went down.

One Sunday my father asked me to print invoices for a client, the Nasipit Lumber Company. As I was printing leisurely, at a pace of 15 paper sheets per minute, the engine went wild. This was very alarming. Something might break and one of the rollers might come off and hit me in the face or my body or neck. I jumped to the gasoline engine, roughly four meters away. As the engine slowed down, the flywheel of the printing press came off its shaft! The steel pin had loosened itself from the main shaft.

That experience made me shake all over for a few minutes. My knees were shaking hard.

The pin had not been checked for many months. The flywheel made a loud bang as it hit the concrete floor. I was on its path! In a tenth of a second or less, I would be smashed. All of a sudden the flywheel swerved to my right side by an inch or two. I felt the wind swish past me. If the flywheel had not swerved to my right it could have crushed me to death. There was no time for me to duck or jump to the other side.

What happened was that when the flywheel came off, it hit the wood that anchored the printing press to the concrete foundation. If this anchorage had been cut a little shorter, like by an inch, the flywheel could have gone straight towards me. I was in luck.

A few months later, the regular printer was routinely running the machine when suddenly the flywheel came off again. It went straight ahead, did not swerve, crashed into the wooden wall, and shattered it. The flywheel almost penetrated the strong wall made of thick timber. To think that the flywheel came off with a normal speed, how much more when it is running three or four times faster when the gasoline engine would rev by itself as it happened to me. Why didn't it swerve? Thank God I was safe when I thought of this incident. It swerved to the right – and avoided hitting me --when I was doing the printing one Sunday.

Was it Lady Luck who protected me from harm when I was operating the printing press a few months earlier and the flywheel came off and swerved to the right?

My father realized the danger posed by a flying flywheel, so after some time he got a new induction motor. From thence the running of the printing machine was smooth, had less noise and never went into unexpected speed again.

THE HOT LAKE THAT
WAS TOO COLD!

A venture I remember very well was when I attended a Christian Young People's Conference (CYF) one summer (1953) in Lake Mainit, Surigao Province, Philippines. "Mainit" means "hot" in the local vernacular. The residents claimed that when the volcano Hibukbihuk (in Camiguin Island) which was 300 miles away erupted in the past, the northern end of the lake would boil, hence the word "mainit" was used to describe the area. This was due to a subterranean connection under the continental shelf.

The last day of the conference was picnic day. The morning was full of splendor. A group of young people hired a motorboat. I joined them but after a few minutes, about a hundred meters from the shore, I decided to jump. I then realized that the water was very cold. After a minute of swimming in this freezing lake water one of my legs went into titanic spasms. I tried to relax and float so as to relax my whole body but I could not. The cold chill in my back muscles sent pains all over my back and down the legs. I felt my abdominal muscles and diaphragm getting very tight. I started sinking! Suddenly, I saw the boat coming back towards me. Someone had seen me and shouted, "He is drowning!" One shouted. The boat swerved towards me. What a coincidental rescue!

The mysterious fact was that the pilot had always been going around the lake clockwise for years to take tourists to some sites. The pilot was amazed. He said he did not know why he turned back, something he did not do before. Was it coincidence? What made him turn back counter clockwise? I leave the matter for you to ponder on.

THE VOICE THAT COMMUNICATED WITH ME

When I was almost 20 years old, I encountered one of the most mystifying experiences in my life at that time. I was in my fourth year in college. At that time, I pretended and claimed I had gained much knowledge in the physical sciences, especially in Paleontology, Comparative Anatomy, and related subjects. As I learned and intellectually acquired more facts, I doubted if believing in religion was right, and the existence of God! I even proclaimed there was no God! Now, I know that the knowledge I had acquired at that time was very meager. Limited knowledge, indeed, can be very dangerous.

I used to discourse with Theology students on sensitive matters. I said, Evolution, not Creation was the truth! I would argue with them, stating scientific facts and discoveries. Darwin's theory really attracted me. (Of course, the process of evolution is true, as scientists have postulated and investigated. The scientists should be credited for their lifework. This is how God created the whole physical Universe and beyond! It was for man to discover His wonders).

I reasoned that religion was a result of man's fears and insecurities so that for comfort, man had to form organizations, secular or political or whatever, within the many human societies in every corner of the earth.

One Saturday morning in 1957 while in my deep slumber in Doltz Hall Dormitory where I was lodging, at about four o'clock in the morning, I was awakened by a voice that seemed to come from a loud speaker. The loud voice filled the room. It was a kind but deep and penetrating voice. And the voice said: **"Thou shall prophesy!"** Whose voice was that? Was I dreaming? I knew I was not dreaming. The voice woke me up from my deep sleep. I asked, "Who is there?"

A cold shiver ran through my spine when I recalled those three words. The words were distinctly clear. Was it a ghost? I could not accept it was an auditory hallucination.

Although I was confused, I convinced myself that it was not the voice of any of my three roommates. It was so different from their voices. I jumped out of bed (the beds were separated by a floor–to–ceiling wall), switched on the light to see if any of my roommates were in their bunkers. Nobody was in! I was alone! None of my three roommates were in their room. They must have gone home to their hometown for the weekend some 50 or 100 kilometers away. I was in a quandary. Did somebody really speak to me?

I took this incident lightly, but as years passed, I kept recalling hearing those three words.

I never discussed the incident with anybody. Nor did I engage myself in conversations about religion and science opposing each again. I tried to reconcile the possibility of science and religion going together. Today, I am convinced that both are compatible. A lot of people take the words in the Bible literally. This is where the conflict and confusion lie.

That experience of hearing the unusual voice and the message disturbed me for a long time, but inspired me to read the Bible more seriously than ever. Nobody knew those words and I kept that a secret for over 50 years.

For a protracted time I wanted to know whose voice talked to me that early morning. Was it the voice of Jesus Christ? Was it my grandfather's? Or was it my imagination? I had to search the psychic world to satisfy my curiosity.

6

LOST IN THE MIST

The summer of 1956 was my first time to join a zoological expedition in Mount Malindang, Zamboanga Del Norte, a province in Mindanao, the second largest island in the Philippines. There were 18 of us in the team organized by Prof. Dioscoro Rabor, head of Silliman University's Biology Department, and his assistant, an instructor at the department. Three members were pre-med students (I was one of them); the rest were regular members of the expeditionary team who had many years of experience collecting mammals of all kinds, reptiles, shooting all species of birds, small or big that crossed their path.

Dr. Rabor and his team did this every summer school break. The expedition would last two months in the rugged mountain areas. The specimens were sent to Chicago Natural Museum. The bird's meat and bones were removed, the skin stuffed and preserved in Borax, then dried in the sun. The specimens collected were for scientific research purposes. The meat was cooked by the chef in the group; his dishes, spiced up with herbs, were delicious.

Many days were spent preparing camping equipment, guns, ammunition, axes, bolos, spades, and food.

The day came for my first participation in the team two days after the end of the school year. All of us were eager to go. We took an inter-island boat with a capacity of 200 passengers but actually had loaded more than 300 on board. It was an old FS used by the Americans after the war. The vessel chugged for ten hours, from Dumaguete to Dipolog, Zamboanga Del Norte.

Most of the time the sea was calm during that season of the year--but not on the day we sailed to Dipolog Thirty minutes in the open sea, I felt nauseated from the endless heaving and swaying of the boat. Then I felt like throwing up. "Will I have enough time to run to the window to throw up?" We were all congested in the lower deck. There was no room to maneuver. The cots were so close to each other that only one of the passenger's legs could pass through the space.

When I was about to spew, I stood up to run to the window with both hands covering my mouth. As soon as I stood up, I felt so sick I had to squeeze my face between two cots and vomited. Almost half of the passengers were seasick, and many vomited on the floor. One could smell the rancid odor all over the place. However, other passengers were heartily eating on the table. They tightly held their plates when the boat rocked or swayed. I wondered why they did not get nauseated or vomit

After hours of that gruelling experience, which seemed endless at the time, we embarked at our destination, and prepared our things for the bus that would take us to a village, Salvacion, some 42 kilometers away. After coming out of the boat, walking on the wharf was like staggering after a heavy bout of alcohol abuse. It felt like the wharf was heaving and swaying as though I was still on the boat. I looked for a place to sit as I felt like vomiting again. I was sweating, cold and weak, from the previous sleepless night. It took more than half an hour before I could walk steadily again. We hired a small bus to take us to Salvacion, the nearest village at the base of Mt. Malindang, the mountain range where we would be collecting all kinds of animal life. It took us a few hours to reach our destination. We settled that night in an empty hut in that village. We were packed like sardines when we went to bed.

The next day, Professor Rabor and two experienced party members went to reconnoiter the area to find a suitable place for a base up in the mountains. When they returned that night, a decision was made on the location of the base camp. This was at 5,000 feet above sea level. We had an altimeter. At least we had a day of rest before our task began.

We set out at five o'clock the next morning as the first streaks of dawn appeared in the horizon. Early start was necessary. It took us seven hours to reach the edge of the forest. Once we had to stop to rest and find a shade as the heat of the noonday sun was merciless. There was very little shade we could take shelter except cover our heads with clothes or raincoats.

We were very far from the forest edge yet. The temperature ranged from 40 to 44 degrees Centigrade (104 to 122 deg. F) from 11 o'clock in the morning until 3 o'clock in the afternoon. The first two hours of hiking with 30 to 40 kilos load or 50 kilos (for the huskier fellows) strapped to our backs seemed easy. Much of the heavier load, like sacks of rice and other provisions for our two month expedition were carried by sleds pulled by a tamed water buffalo.

We went up and down valleys, hills and flat fields. We saw the lofty mountains, actually bluish in color, some ten kilometers away.

At a distance we walked like small ants in a column. Endless minutes passed and the temperature as we walked got even hotter. The heat exhausted me as well as the two other pre-med newcomers, but not the well-trained and conditioned members and the hired locals who helped with the load. During a 20- minute break, some sat on one side of the water buffalo to get shelter from the sun. We wished we had umbrellas. We only had raincoats in our knapsacks.

We saw the base of the tropical forest. It seemed so close yet so far. We had a few more kilometers to walk. To the novice like me, the last few kilometers made me wish I did not join the expedition.

Reaching the forest edge and resting on the cool shade was paradise. Thick underbrush occupied most of the forest floor. Some areas were clear and clean, and the fresh air was different from the smog of the city. It smelled so good. All of us took deep breaths and felt the relaxing effect of the cool breezes. I could not help saying loudly, 'Oh, how refreshing to be here!' Somehow our tiredness seemed to disappear.

Thirty minutes of rest, then the real climb started. Hired farmers now carried the supplies that were placed on the sled. The water buffalo could not do the 45 to 55 degree climb up the mountains. Regular team members had to carry their loads on improvised wooden boxes that were then strapped to the shoulders. The trail was a gradual climb from the base of the mountain where thick tropical rain forests were abundant. At about 2,000 feet above sea level, we would go up a 45 degree climb, so that we were forced to use both hands to pull ourselves up. We climbed ridges, and then ever so gingerly walked down ravines.

I was struggling when we were at about 4,000 feet above sea level. The other pre-med student, Felino, and I almost emptied some of our load and planned to come back for them the following day. After every ten or 15 minute climb we took a 5 minute rest. Felino and I were always at the tail end of the group. The professor was behind us. He was always last of the group, lagging behind intentionally, checking, and limping from a previous injury to his right ankle incurred in an earlier expedition.

The trail was almost invisible as we climbed the last 1,000 feet. We got lost twice. We went back and found twigs pointing at the direction we were to follow.

The others had arrived early at the area where our base camp was to be set up. Tents had been pitched when we reached the place. A few minutes' rest, a cup of coffee and a puff at a cigarette (for the smokers) behind a large tree trunk were like heaven. The professor did not like the smell of cigarette fumes, that's why the smokers had to steal a puff 30 meters away. For non-smokers like me, the air was very soothing to the surface of the skin and lungs. Being in the campsite invigorated us again. The regular team members understood why it took us long to reach them. They teased us as slow folks, but we did not mind, we were newcomers.

At last, we were able to make it to our first day of expedition in these virgin forests! We didn't know that a few months of workouts in the school gymnasium helped condition our bodies for the task that lay ahead.

Dinner was ready before the sun gave up its last streak of light. Somebody lit the kerosene lantern. The camp brightened and we could see the faces of the team members.

The meal was so tasty even though it was plain rice and canned sardines. The atmosphere, the sweet fragrance of the forest and the serenity surrounding us whet up our appetite. We were happy, and at peace.

Darkness settled as the kerosene lantern was turned off. A cool air brought a thick mist into the camp, only to disappear after a few minutes. We were probably above the clouds. Our chubby chef, Minoy, was a musician and singer. He had a nice baritone voice. He started to play his guitar and Sergio, our assistant cook, who played his harmonica, accompanied Minoy when he sang with his guitar. They played familiar tunes. The melodies were pleasant to hear. There were no audible sounds in the stillness of the evening. There was no dashing of the wind but a distant rushing sound of a murmuring brook could be heard. The silence was broken with the fast song of Elvis Presley by one of the boys: 'They call me poor boy, poor boy.' That song was the hit that summer.

It was a pleasant evening

We slipped into our improvised sleeping bags early but I could hardly sleep. Every time I moved, a muscle or joint would ache. The more conditioned fellow with me was deep in slumber like a log. My tent mate would not wake up even if you put a teaspoon of salt in his open mouth. As soon as I dozed off, the professor shouted loud and clear: 'Wake up, everybody! Wake up.' It was still pitch dark. I thought it was the middle of the night. When I glimpsed through the slit in the tent, I saw that dawn had broken!

It was cold! One read the thermometer. 'It's 6 degrees Centigrade!' Everybody had to do something to start work for the day to make his body warm.

The next three weeks were exciting and thrilling experiences. Everyone had a specific task assigned to him permanently for the duration of the expedition. Some had the 8-gauge double-barrel shotgun; others had a 410-gauge shotgun for the smaller birds and .22 dust guns for the tiny birds and air rifles. We had to practice zeroing our rifles.

Every day we shot and collected whatever we could see in the living rain forest, from lemurs to hornbills, to snakes and tree frogs.

There were times I felt pity for the beautiful birds with their beautiful downy feathers, like the Philippine trogon. This is a rare bird found only in that part of the world. A deep sorrow would hit my heart for a fleeting moment. Maybe its partner was looking for him, I would tell myself. I wondered if those birds and animals had souls in them. After a moment, I had to dismiss this notion and not be carried away. I had to do what I was there for. The expedition was for scientific purposes.

At night, two or three guys went hunting for deer. They got lucky occasionally. The venison tasted so good. With this zoological expedition, the abundance of fresh meat was endless. You see, when we skinned the birds we dissected the flesh and bones. In that manner, we were able to taste all kinds of bird meat, from the Monkey Eating eagle to the smallest ground bird, and all kinds of meat of different mammals. Nobody could tell the difference. The herbs and spices served their purpose. We indeed had a very good cook! Sometimes we thought we were eating fowl meat only to be told it was from a monitor lizard. We could not refuse any second serving if there was anything left.

After a week, we started to enjoy the routine, going out early in pairs, taking our lunch boxes, tucking in a raincoat, and a collector's bag with a box of matches in it. The bag was strapped at the waistline to carry the catch of the day. Coming back in the afternoon, we counted our catch. Every week, the fellow who had collected the most number of specimens, especially of birds, would be given a tap on the shoulder.

We collected specimens in the forest floor within a three to five kilometer perimeter of the campsite during the first few days of our expedition. We hunted below and above ridges and peaks, spanning gorges and ravines from eight to 15 kilometers every day, even on Sundays. No day was wasted even on rainy days. Sometimes during the hunt for birds difficulties were encountered. Retrieving a struggling bird after it had been shot could be a difficult task especially when the bird went into hiding under a thick brush or a deep ravine; sometimes the wounded bird was lost forever.

After three weeks, it was time to establish a sub-camp. A possible site had been chosen earlier by the professor in the company of two team members. It was approximately 18 kilometers away, on much higher ground from the base camp. By this time we had collected much of the representative species mostly of birds in the mountain range. Scientific data were entered for every specimen collected, tagged, large or small, weighed, numbered, date of collection, and name of the locality or mountain range.

It took a day to establish the sub-camp. Two boys were left to guard the main camp and at the same time collect specimens for their supply of fresh meat. Their main job was to dry all the specimens in the open when the weather was good and the sun shining. The smaller reptiles and amphibians were preserved in 10% formalin.

At the second camp, everybody had the chance to rotate and stay there at least once a week. The person assigned was responsible for the main meal at night when the hunters came home. He saw to it that the specimens were dried under the sun, and he had the chance to do his laundry in cold water. The soap hardly bubbled when we washed our dirty clothing in hard water.

On my first day as person-in-charge in the sub-camp, I had a horrifying experience. Our camp was at the edge of a clearing some 30 meters near a corner of the thick virgin forest. At about 10:00 o'clock in the morning, a troop of about 50 monkeys (young and old)—the whole tribe, I suppose -- came close to the camp. I was drying skinned specimens that moment. I reached for the double-barreled shotgun, loaded it with the number 8 buckshot, and crept slowly towards the troop. They knew I was there. They were all silent. I just needed one, I thought to myself. I talked to myself that we would have monkey meat for dinner when the party comes home.

These primates were clever! When you look for them with a gun in your hands they would hide and vanish as if the forest was lifeless. I could not detect even a faint of movement in my field of vision. I knew they were hiding behind the trees. I just wanted to get one of them.

I was stalking a big one. There was one that I spotted earlier. He could be the leader of the group. Usually, there is a communal leader, and then the rank and file. If I could get this big one, this would be a prize catch, I told myself. When I spotted and aimed at one of them, all the monkeys seemed to know he had no chance with the gun I had. They all made loud noises as if there were hundreds of them—trying to distract my concentration or to scare me off.

I aimed at the closest. This one had a small one behind her back, one arm clutching the baby monkey, but it was too late! I had pulled the trigger! My God! I got the baby monkey too!

They did not fall.

I knew the mother was wounded with the two-gauge shotgun blast. I used one cartridge. To my surprise she did not fall but then a second or two later—the baby monkey fell to the ground. The mother came down quickly. Before I knew it, the wounded mother was rushing towards me together with two big ones, extremely mad, screaming in their own language, bellowing in anger! I did not have any extra cartridge left. I had only one cartridge, but I had used one the day earlier, and then the second, to shoot at the monkey. I did not have time to reload. I ran as fast as I could back to the main tent to get more ammunition. This was 15 meters away. The mother monkey almost caught my leg when I was near the working tent.

I stopped to face the enemy to defend myself with the handle of the shotgun but she stopped, and so with the other two big ones who followed her. They looked into my eyes with their fierce look, then paused, then retreated slowly. What made them retreat? The mother must have been hit badly. She must be in agony. Why did not the two unwounded monkeys attack me? The monkeys must have been scared too because I was still holding the shotgun. Then the mother monkey that I shot started to show the agony in her face. I could understand and feel a mother's instinct when her young one is hurt or taken away from her. It must be instinct. Of course, the monkeys did not know I did not have any cartridge left. They muttered in their own language as they went back slowly, dejected, to join the other members of the clan. The wounded one showed loss of strength. I could not get ammunition and finish her off.

I was really scared, trembling, and imagined the injuries I could have sustained had the three big monkeys attacked me. With their might and speed, I was surely a goner.

My heart sunk, thinking of the mother's having lost her baby. In fact, there was a strong pity deep in my heart almost to the point of desperation. Since that experience I could not shoot any monkey anymore.

The following day, I had a partner. He was an experienced hunter, having joined the team for more than six years. I thought I had enough experience with the four weeks we had been in the mountain. I suggested we part ways, anyway, the weather was very clear, not a cloud in sight, a perfect hunting day.

I went to a mountain peak where I had been before. This was approximately four or five kilometers from the sub-camp. The top of this particular mountain range was clean with occasional underbrush. The ground was covered with rotting leaves that gave a particular smell of the forest. It was a sweet smell to me. It was not musty. The trees were not very tall. Some trees were flowering and bearing fruit. I knew the birds would come to this area to feed. It was such a good area to stay hidden and wait for the birds to come. I shot the birds down as they came.

In a matter of two hours I was able to get 19 birds of different sizes which I could fully remember to this day. I decided to rest, ate my cold lunch, and took a short nap beneath a shady sub-tropical tree. Before I dozed off I could hear the sound of a shotgun at a distance. That gunshot must have come from my partner -– not so far away.

The nap turned out to be more than an hour instead of a ten-minute break. The chilly air had awakened me. I shivered for a few seconds, looked at my watch: it was one o'clock in the afternoon. It had gotten dark. The mist was thick, and so was the fog that covered the whole mountain. It was clear and sunny an hour ago. I told myself this was probably only a huge cloud that enveloped this mountain range.

Sometimes, from our sub-camp we saw clouds covering this mountain range. After some minutes the cloud would be behind the mountain peak then traversed west. I had hoped the cloud would lift soon or be blown away. It became darker and the mist thickened. The visibility was ten to 15 meters now. Where was the East or West? I had no compass. Which part did I come from? Where was the way to the camp? I could not tell.

My heart started to pump fast! I moved from one corner of the area where I was – 80 to a hundred meters wide -- to look for an exit. I started to panic. Adrenaline was working in my blood stream. I found a small trail. I followed this trail, but it disappeared after half a kilometer run. I should have broken a twig or two before I climbed this mountain range. We usually do this when we come to a new area. Why didn't I? The day had been so clear we could see our sub-camp at a distance. I was there the other day. It was sunny and we knew where we were. Where is my partner? I gave a few calls to my hunting partner. "Are you there?" There was no answer. Has he returned to camp? The forest area looked completely different with the thick mist all over the mountain.

I went back to the top of the mountain again and looked for another trail. Meanwhile the mist got thicker now and the air much colder. I was chilling to my spine. I may not find my way back was in the back of my mind!

I saw another trail. This looked like a man-made trail which local hunters used coming up from the lowlands looking for deer or wild boar. If I could find my way back I should be in the sub-camp in one and a half hours. What if the trail would lead me north or west? I might be going the opposite way. I could be on the other side of the huge mountain range and the nearest village would be 70 kilometers away or more. I would be lost in the darkness when night falls. I decided to follow the trail; I was taking chances. It should take me somewhere. I could not help but run faster and faster down the trail. I never passed this one before! Where would it lead me?

In my haste, I threw my rifle to my right hand or the left so I could cut down the inertia of my flight by grabbing a small tree or branch as I descended the trail. What if the dark night would come soon? I would not be able to move anymore. I had no match in my bag (which we usually carry). I could not start a fireplace to keep me warm through the cold night. Nor did I have extra provisions for my ordeal. I had dead birds in my bag. I could not possibly eat raw meat. My mind went through many things. Would the professor be mad? Will he send a party through the night to search for me? Maybe this is my punishment for killing that baby monkey and possibly the mother monkey, I thought. I prayed in earnest: "Lord, please forgive me for my wrongdoings. Please lead me back to my camp."

It was three o'clock in the afternoon when I looked at my watch again. It felt like I followed a mountain trail that did not lead to the sub-camp and I must have run more than ten kilometers. Despite the rate I was running down, there was no sign of exhaustion in myself. My adrenals were working at high speed. Then I tripped on a large root jutting out from the base of a big tree. I fell forward, accidentally threw my gun a few meters away, and I landed on both wrists. The pain on my wrists was excruciating. "Did I break a bone in my wrist?" When I looked up from the ground, the place looked familiar. I was in our base camp! The site of the base camp filled my heart with excitement. All fears vanished instantly.

I made a triangular run from the sub-camp to the mountain where I got lost. The sub-camp was east of the base camp, about 18 kilometers away. I went up about five kilometers away from the sub-camp and came down west-south-west covering some 23 kilometers.

I could not tell the two fellows who were left guarding the main camp that I got lost! I felt embarrassed! I told them that I was hunting down the trail and decided to pay them a quick visit.

After a few minutes, one suggested that I hurry back to the sub-camp before darkness fell. I borrowed their flashlight. I followed a long, rugged trail, jogging and running on the way back to the sub-camp. Time was running short but my adrenaline kept me going and I made my way back in three hours. The professor was starting to worry and one heard him uttering words hard to describe. You see, sometimes before the sun sets, one got back late, but rarely. Most are back at the camp between four and six o'clock in the afternoon, and in time for the seven o'clock dinner. That was my very first time and last time to be late. Nobody really suspected that I was lost in the mist as I told them I visited the other fellows in the base camp. Nonetheless, I was able to present to Professor my substantial catch of the day.

I learned a lesson that afternoon: one should not break the rule of the expedition. I could have gone to the other side of the mountain and be lost for days.

I had the intuition that somehow *somebody* guided me along the path. You might call this coincidence. There were many coincidental unforgettable happenings in my life, some little things, and some big things that I can't forget.

This experience of getting lost in the mist was one of them.

7

THE STEP TO REMEMBER!

I was 20 years old in pre-medical school.

One particular Sunday morning was splendidly invigorating. I was in a picnic with a few friends at the university farm by the sea. The beach was white, the surf was mild, and the sea was calm. The leaves of tall coconut trees were fluttering in the wind. The heat of the sun was beating on our faces.

Seven of us, all boys, were conversing, sharing jokes and brief stories, at times intently listening to some serious ones. Everybody stood on his ground, not moving an inch for some minutes, maybe an hour. We were in a circle that naturally formed during the conversations. The conversations continued for some time. Suddenly, for no reason, I made one step forward, and all at once, a coconut fell right where I was standing a fraction of a moment earlier. Those who saw this thought it was a miracle. The coconut fruit when it has reached maturity just falls. The coconut above me could have directly hit me on the head had I not moved one step forward at that very instant it fell.

What made me take one step forward? I suppose, my guardian angel could have manipulated a motor center in my brain that made me move without being conscious about it.

Could the mystical world manipulate an accident when the lines hidden in one's palm are written? Some palmists can read the major events as written in one's palm. What about minor events? Where does destiny come in? They say coincidences never happen!

TWENTY FOUR HOURS
OF AMNESIA

This was in my second year in college. We were conditioning ourselves for the next summer expedition at the university gymnasium. We worked on the weights, and occasionally, tried with a pair of boxing gloves. We usually had our workout three times a week for an hour after classes.

One afternoon, a day before our mid-year examination, while we were stretching and warming up with the weights, a classmate invited me to put on a pair of boxing gloves. At first, we threw punches leisurely and before we knew it we were hitting each other with uppercuts, left hooks, and strong jabs with all our strength. I must have hit him with a left cross on his right jaw. This precipitated his anger and gave me a very strong straight blow to my forehead. I could not dock as I was simultaneously giving him a straight into his face. He must have used all his power. This made me stagger!

All I could remember before my right boxing glove reached his face were bright stars for a few seconds. Somebody stopped us as I tried to fight back though in a daze. We made amends, shook hands and forgot the incident.

It was difficult and embarrassing to accept defeat. It had started as a simple, pleasant exercise.

That night I went to bed early, not feeling well. I did not have to review my lecture notes and read my physiology book as I was prepared for the examination the following day.

The following morning, when I sat down for the examination, my mind was completely blank. I could not remember anything of what I had read in my physiology book or learned in class the previous weeks. The questions were strange, as if I had never heard of them before. I could not write any answers at all, nor even dared guess. I took hold of my bearings. I focused on the students around me, the hour, the date, and what happened the previous day. I was totally oriented, except for this amnesia at this particular morning. My mind was completely blank. What will I do? I sat there, pretending to concentrate, hoping that the knowledge I had gained in my studies would return. Perspiration slowly ran down my forehead.

The instructor was at the back of the classroom watching anybody who might be cheating. Apparently, he had been watching me. He must have noticed something was wrong because while others were busy with their pens, I was just holding my pen but not writing anything. He came to me and asked if there was something wrong. I told him that I had a severe headache and I could not concentrate. He could see me off-color and sweaty. He gave me permission to leave and advised me to go to the Out-Patient Department of the University Hospital. I did not go. Instead, I went directly to my dormitory in my bicycle. I had good control of my coordination; I knew the places around me on my way to the dormitory.

I knew it was the blow to my head that caused this amnesia. I might have had a mild concussion. I rested the whole day.

The next morning, I felt fresh. I asked my classmates what were the questions during the examination and I knew the answers. I was ready then to take the special examination the next day.

Since that time I did not put on boxing gloves anymore even for practice sake. I still have this fear (of damaging my brain or the neuronal connections) of losing my memory again – or forever.

9

I ALMOST DROWNED IN
VERY SHALLOW WATER

The second time I joined the Silliman University Zoological Expedition team was in the summer of 1957. Summer school was from the last week of March to the end of May. This was sponsored by Chicago Natural History Natural Museum.

The destination was in the heart of Samar, the locality of Matuguinao. A number of villagers occupied the place at the time. The locale was stunningly beautiful. The mountain ranges were not as lofty as the ones we went to the previous summer. Samar is one of the largest provinces in the Visayas just north of Leyte, the province where Gen. Douglas McArthur first established his beach-head when he "returned" to liberate the Philippines from the Japanese in 1945.

The field work was different from the first expedition in many ways: the scenery, the new faces in the team; the difficult sea travels, the dusty provincial roads, the muddy rugged trails, the unpredictable inclement weather. The kind of forest and the forest floors and their undergrowth, were quite different compared to places we had been to before. The melancholic songs by the group in the night, the occasional burst of laughter by one inside the tent reminded us of the past expedition. And there was the longing for letters from a loved one: but mail at the expedition sites was the same, they were rare: they had to be collected from the nearest post office, which meant a day's hike.

Eight weeks of hard work were delightful and satisfying in this new area. I was always competing with myself, trying to break my own record. I had already a record of 39 birds in one day with a single shot rifle. The record probably must have been broken by now by somebody new in the zoological team.

After four weeks in one area, we all moved and established another camp (not a sub-camp) approximately 20 kilometers away. We brought with us all our equipment and supplies. The first camp was abandoned. I carried a much heavier load than usual to prove to the rest I was strong as anybody else. Essentially, nobody expected everyone to remain in perfect health all the time. I was a small fellow weighing 60 kilos.

The first few hours of walking with a heavy pack ascending hills and descending on valleys was not bad, but by mid-day, exhaustion had overcome me. I let the others go ahead of me.

I tarried longer for an hour after my lunch. We usually ate lunch (in boxes) by ourselves, sometimes with two or three members, if they were around. This time, I ate alone. I was last in the trail. I just felt too exhausted. When I had regained some strength, I lifted the heavy pack to my shoulders.

While crossing a shallow river, mottled by round smooth stones of different sizes, I felt dizzy. I wondered how these round stones were made! Was there a glacier in this area millions of years ago? What I knew was that the main island of the Philippines was connected by a land bridge to Mainland China millions of years ago as evidenced by the same species of pine trees in Benguet province of Northern Luzon, Formosa, and east China.

I looked for the nearest dry spot at the river edge to put my pack in. This was on a sandy dune near the river edge. I tried to unleash my load. Before I knew it, I had passed out for a few seconds or a minute, probably more. I woke up with the right side of my face in the water. If the flowing water was deeper, I could have drowned! The last thing I remembered doing was removing my pack from my shoulders.

I felt so weak again and I walked slowly to a nearby dry area and spread my back flat on dry ground. I must have fallen asleep this time for an hour. When I woke up I felt a trifle stronger. I was not really feeling normal.

When I arrived at the camp, the team members asked why it took me two hours to reach them. I could not tell them that I fainted and almost drowned in shallow water. I told them I was plain exhausted. The professor gave me a tongue-lashing, berating me for carrying a heavy box that should have been carried by the big boys.

The next day looked brighter and I felt sound. We went out in pairs.

As in my first expedition, I and my fellow-hunters oriented ourselves with the new environment. We noted where East or North was situated, studied the mountain and contours which would be our landmarks should we get lost, and got acquainted with man-made trails, rivers and creeks.

By mid-day, on the first hunting day in this new camp, I became lethargic and had a mild chill. I told my partner that I did not feel well. I stayed behind and sat on the hot rocks exposed to the sun. The sun shone brightly, and the atmosphere was hot by any norm yet I felt so cold. After an hour, I dragged myself slowly back to the camp hoping to have enough energy to reach the site. I had collected only five birds, a small jungle lizard and a couple of tree frogs.

Normally, coming back to the camp from the day's hunt, one could tell from the expression on someone's face that his catch was good, fair, or very meager. For the first time, my face showed no life, as if I did not have a collection at all. I told the professor that I was not feeling well.

That night I could only ingest a small amount of food. I had some bad taste in my tongue. I did not have any appetite while others enjoyed their evening meal. I was shivering as I went to bed early. A blanket was wrapped around me -- and to think that the evening was about 30 degrees C. After the chill, I developed high fever. Two aspirin tablets were given to me.

Midnight came. I could hear myself shouting very loudly words out of my mouth, and kept calling the name, "Marcos, Marcos." I was having nightmares! I never had nightmares before. Nightmares are forgotten after a day or so. Somebody shook me. I was half-asleep but I knew what was going on. The fellow sleeping next to me, touched my skin. I was raging with fever!

There was no malaria reported in this area but still we had to take our prophylaxis for malaria once a week. This couldn't be malaria, I thought. What was causing the high temperature? For three days and three nights the fever would not come down. I was thriving only on forced fluids. Did I have a virus? I did not have a sore throat, cough, or joint pains. I only had fever. The professor was getting worried that I might die there in the wilderness and the nearest medical doctor was two days hike away One member of the party had died four years earlier, in an expedition to Mt. Halcon, Mindoro, the second highest mountain peak in the Philippines. That team member died of cerebral malaria.

On the fourth day, my fever subsided during the day but returned in the evening. Our only medicine was aspirin. If this was a virus no antibiotic could kill it. The fight had to be fought by my own immune system. I became weaker and lost some weight. Maybe toxins from the virus or whatever it was that hit me brought down my muscle enzymes. I was so weak that my knees could hardly support me.

The professor was becoming more upset. This would cut short the expedition. They would take me down to the nearest town in another 48 hours if my fever would not totally subside.

On the fifth day, my fever became low grade. I was completely without fever on the sixth day. I noted that on the seventh day I was still so weak I could hardly get up. I remembered my mother, and how she recovered very slowly during World War II.

Convalescence was very slow. I did almost nothing during the last two weeks of this expedition. I was confined to the camp. The professor did not want to take any risk, afraid that I might get a relapse.

Then it was time to fold our tents and move out. We felt sad leaving the place, knowing that we will never return there.

I was much stronger though not one hundred per cent well. Bitterness had clambered into my heart as I felt I was useless during the last three weeks of the expedition. What could I do? It was partly a fault not of my own making.

On moving-out day, I was not allowed to carry anything. The party had made two large bamboo rafts for the whole team and went down the Matuginao River in one day. This was from the center of the province to the eastern shoreline of Samar. It was enjoyable but with some difficulty at times. The nasty rapids were memorably risky, though exciting. We entered the heart of the province coming from the west and came out east.

When we arrived back at the university campus, the Professor asked the hospital authorities to admit me for a thorough investigation. At that time there was an outbreak of the Asiatic Flu. This had been going on for a couple of weeks. Did I have the same virus? It could not be. We were not in contact with civilization for several weeks before the outbreak of the pandemic influenza of 1957.

On the second hospital day, I developed chills, fever, joint pains and severe headaches. I must have contracted the influenza virus possibly from the passengers in the boat coming home because there were passengers who had the flu. As usual, with inter-island vessels, the boat was over-crowded with passengers.

This time I really felt the effects of the influenza virus. Symptoms were totally different from the raging fever I had in the mountains of Matuginao. If it was the same virus I would have developed immunity to this Asiatic Flu. What was the cause of the fever? Doctors would call it today, FUO – or fever of unknown origin.

Everybody in the team remained in good health throughout the pandemic season. Why was it only me who developed this fever of unknown origin? I lived another day to tell the tale.

10

A STRANGE CLOUD FORMATION

D r. Lawrence Q, an entomologist from Bishop Museum, Hawaii, was introduced to me to collect insect specimens with him in the vicinity of Mt. Canlaon located in the center of Negros Occidental, a province in the western Visayas. This was under the sponsorship of the US Navy at that time. Mt. Canlaon is the third highest mountain peak in the Philippines.

I was recommended to Dr. Q. by the Professor, head of the Department of Biology, Silliman University, because I had experience in collecting animal species and I could interpret the local vernacular. Aside from that, I was majoring in Biology and entomological exposure would add to my experience.

The meeting with Dr. Q. was a prelude to my collecting insect specimens the next five summers. My earnings from these entomological expeditions would help me financially through medical school. Without those summer jobs, I would not have been able to go to the University of the East Ramon Magsaysay Medical Center in Manila.

The view from Mr. Canlaon, an extinct volcano, was splendid. The main crater at 8,220 feet above sea level, the highest point, was still spewing with thin fumes. The last eruption was in 1908. South of this crater, 500 meters away was a flat field, three times the size of a football field. A week later, I went down to this extinct crater which is now filled with soil. It resembled a flat soccer field though much larger. The thought of being in that beautiful verdant field was very inspiring.

There were three of us in this entomological party. We hired local hands to guide us and carry our provisions for ten days. We set up camp at the forest edge at 6,000 feet altitude.

From that level, the mountain was bare up to the crater. We saw nothing but huge rock boulders, stones of contrasting sizes, and coarse sand in between ledges.

The first few days, we collected all forms of insect life with butterfly nets around the margin of the forest below our camp. We set up light traps at night to attract nocturnal insects. The specimens were arranged one by one inside boxes, the larger specimens in large boxes, and the smaller and fine ones in pill boxes, layer by layer, separated by a soft material. The pill boxes came in varying sizes. We arranged the catch meticulously as soon as we were back in the camp. Dr. Q. would stay late in the evening until every specimen was in properly contained in white cardboard containers. He called them pill boxes.

As soon as daylight broke we collected the light traps filled with specimens of moths of different varieties and other winged creatures of the night.

The light trap consisted of a kerosene lantern (Petromax) that burned overnight or until the fuel was consumed. A large funnel was connected at the bottom of the lantern where a bottle containing cyanide was placed underneath a trimmed cardboard. This protected the evaporation of cyanide powder. The fumes of the cyanide killed the insects as soon as they fell into the trap. The upper surface of the cardboard would lay all kinds of specimens during the night.

The wind became perky and nasty on the eve of Christmas. We hated this altitude when the wind blew strongly. The chill factor probably dropped below zero. Our teeth chattered even with the glowing amber from the logs we burned earlier. Dr. Q felt cold too despite the fact that he came from a temperate country. We faced the heat from the burning logs but our back would freeze. We turned around after a few minutes and faced the burning logs. Dr. Q. was well equipped with winter clothing, but not the two of us. At eight o'clock that cold windy eve of Christmas, there was no alternative but crawl early into our sleeping bags.

Dr. Q. wished us all: "Merry Christmas Eve!"

On Christmas Day, 1958, we decided to explore the crater. It was still windy and cold. It took us two hours to reach and view the crater, ninety to a hundred meters in diameter, slightly oval in shape. The inner rim of the crater was a vertical drop. I crouched at the very edge, and sensed as though the crater would pull me into its mouth. I felt the volcano swaying. It must have been my balancing equilibrium that made me feel that way. I could not stand at the rim. A sudden blast of strong wind could push me into the crater. Falling was a shuddering thought. I threw a rock the size of my fist. I could hardly hear the sound of the rock hitting the bottom. I could hear the whistling hollow sounds when a strong wind passed by as if one was blowing the mouth of an empty bottle. I threw more rocks and heard the echoing sounds ten or 12 seconds later. It must be more than 500 below or more. We could only guess. Was it solid rock below? I could not guess.

It was mid-day, Christmas Day, and we spent 30 minutes appreciating the magnificent view of the lowlands. We could see east and west of the whole province of Negros Occidental; the shores loomed faintly below and were a little blurry. The air around us was coated with a thin mist. It seemed the shores were just below our feet but they could be more than 200 kilometers away.

After moments of silent appreciation of the beauty we saw we proceeded to the old crater.

At the rim of the dead crater were dwarf sub-temperate trees eight to ten feet tall. We collected varieties of insect forms in our paths or whatever we could reach and scoop up with our butterfly nets. Most of the surrounding areas in this extinct crater had thick undergrowth, and swinging our butterfly nets was impossible. We simply swung our nets in open spaces above the grass and dwarf trees. We were able to collect the tiniest of insects, tinier than a pinhead.

As I was collecting along the sides, I found a boar's trail that led to the field below. I was separated now from Dr. Q. I saw him clearly waving at me with his butterfly net. He was collecting around the border at the other side while I was already in the open flat field. He probably could not find an entrance to the open field as the bush was very thick. I thought he wanted to come down too to this huge "football" field.

Standing in the midst of the field, so even and smooth, was captivating. The field was covered by a fine Bermuda-like grass spread out smoothly. It felt so solemn and mellow while looking up the sky. If it had rained heavily there would be a lake. There was no outlet where the water could flow out. There was no way to tell. Somewhere must be an outlet if rain flooded the area. Otherwise this would be a beautiful lake.

I could hear faint hollow sounds when a gust of wind and clouds rolled over with an enchanting tune at a distance. The enchanting sound must have been created by the wind as it crossed the crater. And then suddenly, from nowhere, *one huge cloud seemed to settle in the wide field, its lower portion dancing with the music!*

This presented a magnificent display. It was almost magical! What was going on? The huge cloud split into two. This cloud should have rolled away as the air current was strong. No, it did not! For a few minutes, it was dancing, right before my eyes, and then gradually rolled on. The scene reminded me of the movie "The Ten Commandments" when Moses split the Dead Sea and the water looked like waterfalls on both sides. It was almost the same picture as the movie. What a remarkably breathtaking scene to behold! Everything around the place seemed alive! The air current must have done that, I suppose. Or did it? After some time all the clouds vanished.

After an hour I met Dr. Q. at the ridge. He was feeling cold.

'Did you see a mass of clouds that gathered in the field?' I asked Dr. Quate. 'No,' he answered, and added, 'I saw you clearly like an ant in the center of the green field swinging your butterfly net back and forth.'

It was strange that Dr. Quate did not see any hovering clouds over the field. Was it my imagination? If it was not my imagination why was it shown to me? Maybe he was too busy collecting bugs to notice the clouds hovering and presenting a magnificent display.

It was two o'clock in the afternoon when we started coming down to the camp. Dr. Q. and I split ways, collecting any bug that we could spot along the way. He went west of the crater and I went down east, towards our camp. I felt cold and hungry, and the wind was blowing stronger than ever. The north wind was even stronger. I did not know why I felt so cold when I was burning with energy. As I was coming down between two huge boulders, my hand touched the huge rock on the right. It was hot compared with the one on the left side. Beside the hot rock was a small opening that was throwing up steam. One could cook an egg in one minute in the super-hot steam. I figured the opening must be connected to the boiling lava trapped underneath the inactive volcano. I leaned back on the hot rock and felt cozy and warm. I fell asleep for half an hour and dreamed of that beautiful cloud formation, splitting, dancing in front of me with a strange melody behind it.

The magnificent sight kept lingering in my mind that night. Why was I shown that amazing cloud formation? I wonder if others who had come to that field before had ever seen one like it.

Was this a manipulation from the mystical world?

11

BLESSING FROM ABOVE!

I finished Pre-Medical School in March 1959 and had earned a Degree of Science, Major in Biology. Usually, after two years of pre-medical courses (with the Title of A.A., Associate in Arts) one can go to proper medical school. In my case I decided to have the four-year course so that if I failed to go to medical school, I could teach in any high school or even in a University. There was that extreme fear I could not really finish medical schooling knowing the very poor financial situation of my family. My father was somewhat hesitant to send me to medical school because he knew too well that my IQ was just average and his financial resources were meager. He said doctors should have very high IQ. He doubted if I could cope with the studies in Medicine. If I did not finish, it was a waste of time and money.

The Philippine school summer holidays of 1960, April and May, was my first time to lead my own entomological expedition of four members. Two were my two younger brothers, Lemuel, and a cousin.

Bishop Museum of Hawaii, U.S.A., financed this expedition through the help of Dr. Lawrence Q and Setsuko N. Bishop Museum used to be under the management of the US Navy. (My wife and I went there in 2006 hoping Dr. Q. and S. N were still alive. Bishop Museum was no longer connected with the US Navy.) Without this summer work, I would not have been able to proceed to medical school. This work was the major source for my tuition fees and lodging expenses during the next five years of schooling. I was very grateful to them and the US Navy.

12

A HUGE TREE FELL ON OUR CAMP!

My first entomological expedition in April 1960 was in the mountain ranges of Misamis Oriental, my home province. This summer was full of experiences quite different from the zoological expeditions I had joined the previous years.

Forty kilometers west of my hometown, is a mountain range that extends to Bukidnon Province. The province is almost at the heart of Mindanao. Mindanao is the second largest island in the Philippines located in the southernmost part of the country. It had virgin forests untouched by advancing civilizations except for a few friendly nomadic tribes that still exist today.

We hired a jeep and followed an abandoned road 35 kilometers inland from my hometown. Logging companies had created the roads, immediately after the Second World War. Most of the tall trees were gone, except those areas inaccessible to men carrying logging equipment. Areas cleared by logging have been settled by farmers. Areas not claimed by farmers were reforested.

It was difficult to get rides during those days. We made boxes with improvised thick straps from conveyor belts and packed our equipment and provisions in wooden containers. At the end of the road where the jeep we hired stopped and could not move further. We fastened the load to our backs and started the trek looking for a place to set up our camp. After four hours of walking in this not so barren terrain we found the area suited for our kind of work.

Around the vicinity were semi-nomadic tribes, the men still wearing G-strings that covered their private areas. Their forebears had been wearing G-strings for centuries. The women had bare breasts, and a piece of rotting cloth around their private parts and loins.

There were some who did not wear G-strings anymore but short pants. Their children wore T-shirts which probably had never been washed since they were acquired. The shirts were so dirty with multiple holes in them. The younger ones did not wear short pants but were bare in the lower half of the body. The older ones had torn garments that served the purpose of covering their delicate parts.

We camped at a secluded place in a gorge. There was a small waterfall 15 meters west of our tents. From a high rocky cliff flowed small waterfalls 20 feet high. North of us was a high mountain range sheathed by a thick rain forest, and south, an elevated ground covered by monocot sharp-bladed plants. All these acted as windbreaker during windy days. East was farmland planted to coffee plants, corn and root crops by farmers. The water source was a brook just a few meters from our tents. The water was crystal clear.

We erected our working and sleeping tents on the north bank of the brook. On the other side was our kitchen where we cooked and stored our food supplies. We chopped firewood for our cooking. The kerosene stove we had was used only during rainy days. To cross the shallow brook, we placed flat stones arranged for the purpose. We ate anywhere. Sometimes on a rock beside the brook or an exposed root of a huge tree, or on the portable table in the working tent. It was picnic day most of the time whenever we had meals in the camp. We enjoyed being in the surrounding wilderness, attaching ourselves to nature. Sometimes the tropical rains marred the day but there were always plenty of things to do.

We had an intelligent dog with us, named Phil. He was a good companion and we had lots of fun with him.

One morning, when my cousin Ingo, was fixing our breakfast, the brook swiftly rose and water was everywhere, flooding the kitchen, and carrying away the stock of firewood. The pot of rice that was still simmering was almost dragged by the flash flood had it not been anchored to the tripod made of wood. It was not fun at that moment but after a couple of days we were laughing as we talked about how we all panicked and ran as fast as we could to save our personal belongings and the kitchenware from being carried away by the water.

Thirty minutes earlier, it had rained heavily a few kilometers above our camp, but not a drop of rain fell on us. Then, to our surprise, the brook suddenly became a flooded river. Ingo had to finish cooking on the kerosene stove.

Above us, roughly 150 meters high, where the source of the small waterfall appeared, was a small clearing. A farmer had felled the tropical trees. That was supposed to be illegal. We went up to this clearing above us and saw the trees that had been felled a few months earlier. We could tell, because the fallen trees were not too old. The farmers would plant crops, rice or corn in this clearing, but there were no crops planted yet. In a few months, whoever cut down the trees would burn the tree stumps in the clearing which we call locally as *"kaingin"*. They burn these cleared areas when the branches and leaves have dried. Because the bigger trees had been cut, rainwater flooded freely down the clearing, swelling the brook, and running down to our camp.

There was a nasty rumor spread among the local inhabitants in the nearby farm areas that we were soldiers belonging to the Philippine Constabulary dressed in civilian clothes and that we were pretending to be insect collectors but actually wanted to catch illegal *kaingeros*. What a destructive rumor! This rumor irked the farmers around because most of them were guilty.

One morning as the day brightened, we heard the distant sounds of a tree being cut down. We concluded that they came from a far distance. It reminded us of the same sounds we heard the day before,--and that was late afternoon--when someone was really cutting a tree. That early morning we thought the person who was cutting a tree with his sharpened axe was finishing his illegal work.

Normally, as soon as I woke up, I did my usual work of arranging insect specimens in pillboxes. These were caught by the light trap set during the night. The boys prepared breakfast or washed their dirty clothes or played with Phil.

That early morning, while placing the catch of the night into the pill boxes, I heard a sudden rustling sound. At that moment, Ingo was brushing his teeth near the tent. A huge tree, about 50 meters long, was coming down on us so abruptly! In a split second, we all could have been dead, But, wonder of wonders, the tree somersaulted in the air as it was falling down on us. Its sharp trunk which was more than a meter in diameter, dug into the ground, a foot away from the tent, and just inches away from cousin's feet while he was brushing his teeth. All he could say was "oops!" in a joyful manner while the brush was still in his mouth.

This came so suddenly like a flash of lightning. The lower branch of the tree (the size of my neck) halted just a foot in front of me. It had stopped suddenly as the main trunk had dug into the ground where my cousin was standing. Had it gone a little further my neck would have been instantly cut off? Or if the whole tree had not rolled over and directly fell on our camp we could have all perished. It was a miracle that the tree flipped on its branches. We did not think at that moment that it was a miracle that nobody was hurt! Even the dog, Phil, could not make a sound. The dog must have been very scared.

We came to think a few minutes later that somebody tried to murder us! This was a pre-meditated act! The few farmers around knew where we were situated. Immediately after breakfast, we went up to the clearing where the tree came from and saw the fresh stump. Analyzing the fall of that tree and how it was cut, anybody could tell that it was meant to fall on our camp. It was intentional!

Ingo tucked in the .45 German Luger pistol and we all went up the clearing.

After reaching the clearing and seeing the stump we went to the nearest farmhouse, about a kilometer away. We believed that he owned the kaingin or clearing above us.

'Where is the man of the house?' Ingo asked.

'He is not in,' the woman who stood at the door answered. We believed she was the farmer's wife.

The wife and the two children were frightened. We could sense the husband was around hiding. Ingo showed the gun in his waist and asked if we could buy some chicken as our provision was getting very low. Suddenly, in front of our eyes, **about half a dozen chickens in front of the house twisted their necks and died instantly.** Nobody was even close to the chickens. Was that a plague? What kind was it? It appeared as if somebody invisible was twisting the necks of the chickens. We could see the heads turning backwards 360 degrees, and after one or two seconds, they just dropped dead! **It was so strange**!

Was this strange happening supposed to stop us from doing harm to the fellow? What else could it be?

Anyway, we went back to the camp with a few hens freely given! We forgave the premeditated act.

We never heard anymore of anyone chopping trees since that incident. Did the farmer tell the others what happened to his chickens?

It was later rumored that I was the son of the woman councilor. My mother was well known in the barrios for teaching girls dressmaking in her school.

We kept this incident to ourselves. **We believed that only the mystical world saved us from harm. Was an extraterrestrial behind this episode? Or a guide beyond the extraterrestrial realm? This was one of the most unforgettable experiences we had.**

We did not want to retaliate. No one was hurt anyway.

13

PHIL SAVED MY LIFE!

The first entomological expedition I led was a memorable adventure.

Phil, an intelligent dog that belonged to my family, was lovable. His whiskers and facial expression resembled an Irish wolfhound. His curly coat was like that of a Gordon Seller with a few large black spots in a drab white background. He was proud and showed his chest off when he did a good turn or when he was appreciated.

The first time we went up the mountains, Phil kept some distance ahead of us, most of the time acting as a scout. He would bark, jump, and eagerly run up the trail while we strained ourselves with our load along the trail. He sat on his haunches on an elevated mound looking at us, then jumped away when he saw us approaching.

As we trudged on, we heard Phil barking vigorously. He was not in distress, but wanted our attention. When we saw him, he was fighting a large venomous snake. He tried to seize the snake's tail. The snake would strike at the dog, but miss his target by an inch, and then retract.

Phil's reflexes were really fast. The snake, like a rattle snake, struck at Phil a few times but missed the canine all the time. Phil was driving away the snake from our path! He could sense danger. What a dog! We wondered how Phil could tell a deadly one. By the time we were very close to Phil, the snake slithered into a bush. We patted Phil's head and embraced him to show our appreciation. He wagged his tail, accepting our grateful appreciation, then proudly walked away.

A few days passed after the huge tree fell on our camp. As I came out of my tent, fresh from a deep slumber, I saw Phil at my working table. I got mad because all the pill boxes and the specimens were all over the place. I got hold of a long piece of wood and hit him terribly hard on the back. I could not control my temper. My adrenal glands pumped adrenaline that made me extremely angry. Phil bellowed a real agonizing cry. Slowly, while moaning, he went to a corner by a large tree trunk, curled his body, and placed his chin on one of his forelegs. He looked at me in agony. He suffered. He knew I was angry. He could sense. He understood he had done something wrong.

I picked up all the things, pill boxes, instruments and specimens, while looking at Phil with anger in my eyes. All the hours wasted placing all those specimens in pill boxes! The very fine specimens were too small to be retrieved. The tiny specimens were even smaller than the head of a pin (that you place in a pin cushion).

Phil saw my deep breathing and the expression in my face. He knew I was holding my temper not to hit him again. For an hour, he curled beside a tree, not moving an inch, feeling miserable and cold. His eyes were fixed on me whenever I moved. He thought I was going to hit him again.

Of course, everybody was awakened by the commotion made by the loud howling of Phil. My brother, started to cook breakfast in our improvised kitchen across the brook. My cousin hung up his washing. My other brother, the younger brother, talked to Phil. He was comforting Phil. Nobody talked to me. They knew the mood I was in.

We had coffee and thick pancakes for breakfast. Usually, when we had breakfast, Phil would be full of spirit moving around, wagging his tail and wanting to have his share right away, licking at everybody's hands pleading for a share if there was something left from our ration. He seemed hungry all the time.

I did not give him anything to eat for breakfast. I looked at him a few times, and his gaze was directed at me. He sat at the foot of the tree for almost an hour. His face looked very sad and pitiful. Only his eyeballs moved when I moved around. I wondered if he could read my mind as I could read his.

After breakfast, we started to get ready for the day's work. No food was given to Phil. Phil knew it. He could neither come with us collecting nor joyfully guiding us that day.

Two hours after I hit Phil in the back, we were about to leave camp for another venture. Each one of us had a water canteen tucked to his belt, and carried a butterfly net. A lunch box was wrapped tightly with old newspapers, and placed in the collection bag with a bottle of potassium cyanide.

Phil just sat watching us. He would be alone in the camp.

Unexpectedly, I pitied Phil. I was cruel! I asked Warto to give him food, but Phil would not touch or smell it. Phil kept looking sadly at me.

'Come on Phil, eat this,' but Phil did not move. My cousin tried. My brothers tried. They all failed to appease him.

He maintained his stand, his jaw resting on his paws as if he wanted to say, please forgive me for disturbing the table or was it that he wanted forgiveness from me for hitting him hard? Perhaps he could communicate with me with this kind of behavior. I was touched by his almost human reaction. He was hurt like a little child. Phil could see the thin film of tears in my eyes. It seemed he had tears too.

'Come Phil,' I said, waving at him to come to me, and slowly he got up from his corner and walked towards me. He was hesitant, uncertain, but he obeyed me. I bent my knees and cuddled him. Phil understood my warm embrace. His tail started to wag again. Soon after, he went to eat his food. Phil felt forgiven.

Attired in our collecting gear, we walked towards a trail that would take us towards the clearing above. Phil sat on his haunches, waiting for my command to lead the way. Under those large tropical trees was undergrowth. Smaller trees were concentrated on the forest floor, so thick that the rays of the sun could not penetrate the leaves. Some places under the tropical trees had very little illumination.

About 20 meters from the camp, Phil started to bark continuously as if something was wrong. I paused and turned my head towards the dog. Phil ran towards me. When I was about to move forward, a viper was in front of my face, nearly 18 inches away—ready to strike at my face! This was a deadly viper. We did not have anti-venom. Phil was silent. He knew that I saw the snake. He had warned me! Everyone saw the green viper camouflaged among the green leaves and branches of the underbrush. A hasty move could make the viper strike. Even Phil did not bark. He knew I had to get away from this danger.

I looked at the snake and it looked at me intently. Its eyes were hazel in color. The skin was mottled green. I withdrew very slowly backwards, inch by inch, almost unnoticeable. Time stood still. I could hear the beating of my heart. When I was a meter away I felt safe. The snake and I had crossed paths by chance, neither one of us meant harm. We let the snake go. If this were a zoological expedition, that snake would be in a bottle of formalin.

What intrigued me was the barking of Phil that made me pause. Had I not stopped at that distance, I would have been dead. Thanks to Phil. I knew I was always looking at the ground, taking care not to step on a piece of rock or a prominent exposed root of a tree or looking for a bug that was crawling along the way, but because I was curious about the barking of Phil, I stopped. That very second I stopped, my eyes were on level with the snake's head. Phil's barking – his way of warning me about a deadly snake ready to attack me – saved me. Phil was really more than man's best friend; he was my best friend.

What made Phil bark? Did he see the snake? This was possible.

Phil saved my life! To think that I had really hurt the dog a couple of hours ago, still he warned me of extreme danger.

Pets or any other tamed animals can easily forget hurts, compared with some folks in our world today.

14

FRESH MEAT, A BLESSING!

Another strange circumstance happened in the summer of 1960 when we camped by the bank of a brook. I was heading my own private entomological expedition, or, simply put, insect collection enterprise.

One afternoon, we went down to a farm roughly ten kilometers from our camp to buy fresh meat. We had hoped for any kind of meat that was available from the farmers' backyard poultry or pig farm. In due time, farmers around the area gradually knew who we were. The farmers grew crops, coffee and a variety of vegetables. They also had poultry and pigs in their backyard to sustain their family in comfort. The excess was sold or bartered.

The farmer we knew well in this village of Bal-ason had half a dozen adult pigs and a few piglets. We intended to sleep in his bamboo house that night with his wife's approval. They were always accommodating people and happy to render help in any form once they knew you.

While we were having sips of gin toned by coke, I asked the farmer which pig he would butcher in the morning. The biggest was my choice, I said, pointing to the largest one.

'No,' the farmer said with emphasis. 'That one is for a very special occasion.'

Out of nowhere I said jokingly 'When we wake up in the morning that pig will be mine.'

At daybreak, the pig was dead. It must have died of something we did not know--a few minutes earlier as the blood was still warm. Did the pig have a heart attack? Do pigs get heart problems? In due time, the other pigs would get the virus if there was a contagious disease. This never occurred.

The farmer could not believe it. I told him the night before that that pig was my choice. *Was this coincidence?* **Strange, but it came true.**

And so, we took fresh meat back to the camp.

(Years later I received an Entomology journal that said two species of earwigs were named after my name collected from this particular locality).

15

STUNNED FOR MINUTES!

Our next entomological expedition was in Mount Iriga, Camarines Sur. After 4 weeks, we went to another province, Albay, to look at the famous Mayon Volcano, famous for its perfect cone-shape.

To view the perfect cone with a camera one had to stand 60 kilometers away from the base or from the City of Legaspi. However, when we camped at the base of the volcano at about 2,500 feet elevation, the terrain was utterly rugged.

There was a "Look-out" area where tourists can come closest to the volcano. We were camped about two kilometers away from the area. The trees around were only 10 to 12 feet tall, dense, and which we could hardly penetrate except through small trails. Thick and thorny underbrush filled the lower sides of the volcano. There were man-made trails, almost invisible, which visitors can use if they decide to go up the crater. The upper half of the volcano at 3,000 feet and above was barren. The old road that was created decades ago had been covered by thick bushes, mostly by a tall monocot or *cogon* growth with razor-sharp-edged leaves. This was the first time and place I saw this kind of monocot plant.

The ravines, which were not visible from afar, were deep and largely irregular, forming the cliffs and gorges.

The elevation of the volcano was over 7,000 feet above sea level. The last time it erupted was in 1950. The local inhabitants claimed it erupted every ten years. But the deadliest eruption was about 100 years ago and covered the town of Cagsawa with boiling lava. We could still see the steeple of the church which was buried under solid rocks (molten lava that had solidified). It was midnight when it suddenly erupted. A number of inhabitants of the barrios below the volcano fled that night to the church building, but all the same, nobody escaped from the inferno.

Some areas on the upper half of the volcano were smooth. They were filled with very fine brown sand. The sand was finer than that we walked on the seashore. Our heels could dig in a few inches deep. Some portions were irregularly shaped solid rocks and pebbles in contrasting dimensions.

We collected specimens around the base for a couple of weeks. Afterwards we made a sub-camp at 4,000 feet above sea level, just at the edge of the forest. From there it was all barren up to the top.

After a week in that sub-camp, we decided to clamber up to the crater. The older brother of my cousin, was a tall and hardy companion. He lived in Iriga.

We climbed slowly the next thousand feet, collecting minute insect specimens. A few insects were beneath rocks and crevices.

There were areas where molten lava had flowed and formed rocks with small pools on their top that were filled with water during the rainy season. We tasted the remaining water. It was awful, unlike the spring water below. This was for the birds to quench their thirst.

We thought we could climb the summit in two hours but three hours had passed and we were still climbing. The climb became stiffer, more angled as we were near the top. We calculated the elevation to be about 6,000 feet.

Clouds gathered. They were blown away after a few minutes. The view of the lowlands from this elevation was imposing. The valleys and fields were grayish and the deep blue ocean of the Pacific was grand. We saw the breaking of the surf, below us, that looked like fine froth. The fields and ocean seemed very near. Sitting on a flat rock for several minutes, meditating and looking at the view below, made us feel peaceful. Such a breath-taking panorama! To see such beauty and feel the peace made us wish we could live there forever. But we could not tarry long. We had to keep on.

Mid-day, and four hours had gone. We sensed we were about 200 feet below the crater. The climb was petrifying. The slope had become vertical. We had no ropes for anchor except the butterfly nets that we used to prop or support us between ledges. This was rock climbing using our hands and feet. If we fell nothing would hold us back. We never expected this and were not prepared for this. Still, we continued to climb another hundred feet and we figured we should be at the top in 30 minutes, looking down everywhere, from east to west from north to south. It would be a splendid sight to remember!

Two meters away, as I was wedging myself between two boulders, pushing myself slowly upwards, I saw a rock the size of my head coming down towards me. That rock must have dislodged itself. There were no tremors. Maybe the strong wind did it. If I ducked my hands would probably slip and I could roll down 3,000 feet. I let the rock hit my chest as I gave all the strength I had to push the huge boulders between me so the rock won't dislodge me. The rock bounced off my chest and rolled down the space between my chest and the solid wall in front of me. Thank God it did not hit my face or head. I could have sustained a laceration on the face or my scalp! Or disloged me from my strong hold betwen rocks. The rock rolled on, gathering momentum, and multiplying in number as it hit bigger rocks along its path until we could no longer see them. We hoped the rocks would not reach our camp. A cloud of dust formed broadly at the base near our camp. We heard the distant crashing of rocks against the trees below.

After that, I rested for a few minutes to ease the tension in our leg muscles. Irritating fumes hovered around us. This was sulphur! We did not make a move but stayed another few minutes. Then we noticed that our skin had become pale yellow -- even the white of our eyeballs. Surely we could not have contracted hepatitis to make us look pale-yellowish. But we looked jaundiced! Later the fumes and mist disappeared.

Two jet planes passed. We waved with our butterfly nets. They were gone in a very short time.

I looked at his white eyeballs. They were yellow now, as our skin had turned yellow. Our skin had turned yellow too. We were alarmed. If we stayed longer more sulfuric fumes would be in our system. We decided to climb down as the discoloration became more prominent every minute we stayed longer.

Suddenly, I felt very cold. A strong gust of cold wind made us shiver.

We felt bad because we were not able to look down into the mouth of the crater. The hollow whistling sound a few meters above us gave us the impression that the crater was just above us. We almost made it if not for the sulphuric fumes. These could have poisoned us or possibly precipitated acute bronchospasm to both of us. We had heard stories about people dying around this summit, near the crater a few years ago while climbing the volcano. Could they have been affected by the fumes?

Climbing down the vertical wall, with the butterfly net in one hand, was not easy. Our knees rattled. One false step in our rubber shoes, and it would have been our end. We dared not look down, for the sight of the steep gorge would make us nervous. Sounds were heard in our abdomen as we did not have our lunch yet.

After that most dangerous descent, the rest of the time going down the volcano was very easy and enjoyable. We took our lunch. A few minutes later we slid down the soft sand dunes in between large furrows, and avoided stepping on pebbles and small rocks. Sometimes sitting or standing, we skated down the slopes, using our tennis shoes to dig into the sandy soil for brakes when we went fast. It was fun! But this did not last long.

To control our descent, we used the wooden handle of the butterfly net. The steel ring was clipped under our armpit. We imagined ourselves to be skating on snow. It was a treat for us. What took us three hours to climb up the slope took us only 15 minutes to climb down.

Before I realized it, I could not control my descent. I went so fast — pushed by the inertia of my descent and pulled by gravity so that I could not stop myself. Dust formed behind me and rocks came down racing with me.

My cousin was about a thousand feet above, looking steadily at me, something dreadful was happening! He could not do anything but watch. He could perceive I was in trouble.

I went faster and faster. I tried to dig my heels into the sand as deep as I could and my butterfly net handle as well. The inertia was just so strong; I was splashing the sand sideward as if I were on a water ski.

Sliding down fast, my body was almost parallel to the sloping ground at 35 degrees. I raised my face and neck slightly from the ground so I could see what was ahead of me. A little sway and my body would spin and be gone forever.

I saw a ravine about 50 meters below me. I was heading towards it. I could not swerve to the right otherwise I would just roll and spin downwards. Tony just watched me, hopelessly holding his breath.

Barely two meters away from the edge of the ravine, my heels and the handle of the butterfly net simultaneously hit a rock. This rock stopped me suddenly! If I had not assumed a lying position, the sudden jolt would have thrown me forward and I would have landed a thousand feet below. **This was a miracle to me!**

For a few minutes I was dumbfounded. I thought I was a goner. I could be reported to the authorities as an accidental death! I wonder what really killed the previous climbers. Was it the sulphuric fumes? Or was it their coming down, as what almost happened to me?

I looked back and saw that my cousin was still standing on the slope. He saw everything that happened to me. Then he started to ease himself down the slope.

For a few minutes, my mind was stunned!

I could only thank silently my mystical guide or guides.

16

FLASH FLOODS IN MOUNT ISAROG!

Unlike the mountains in Mindanao and other parts of the Philippines which I had visited, Mount Isarog, Camarines Sur, was not densely covered by tropical rain forest. A road climbed 4,000 feet above sea level to a transmitter site. A VHF station relayed most military and government communications from the southern part of the Philippines.

We camped at 3,000 feet above sea level beside a river. The water was crystal clear. We built a pipeline out of split bamboo that carried water to our tents. To take a swim and clean ourselves from the day's perspiration, we dove into the deeper portions of the river below the camp.

A huge rock, flat and smooth with some mild depressions on its surface lay in the middle of this river. This was around 4 sq. m. in area, big enough for our work table. It was about two meters above the rushing water. What a creation of nature! And it was lovely and cool under the shade of a canopy. The sounds of the mildly rushing water had a soothing effect. There must have been a lot of positive ions in the air to give this soothing feeling. The forest around was invigorating. It was quiet most of the time, except for the occasional bird calls, and the croaking of frogs. On hot mid-days and afternoons, the continuous high pitched sounds of cicadas could be heard everywhere. I had not heard so much cicada noise in the past as in this place.

One Sunday, I stayed in the camp while the boys went down to town, 12 kilometers away. They bought cigarettes and had a few sips of the local rum.

I was routinely arranging the specimens caught by the light traps the night before. It was about one o'clock in the afternoon. Suddenly I heard a loud noise as if a plane was going to crash.

I looked around me and my heart beat faster, alarmed by the strange noise. As the noise came closer, I became more scared. I never heard anything like it in my life! I could not see anything that would cause the distinct unusual sound! In a matter of seconds the strange sound became louder and louder. It came from the mountains just above our camp!

'Is a landslide coming down?' A thought swept into my mind. The noise become louder, and in an instant I saw 15 meters away, a huge flash flood, rising almost three meters high!

The water rushed towards my working tent with a tremendous roar. It had rained heavily 30 minutes earlier somewhere up in the mountains but not in our encampment. It was summer and usually we did not have rains in this part of the archipelago at this time of the year.

My working tent was in its path! I should have known better before I chose this site as my working place. It was too late! Should I jump or stay? I made the decision in a split second.

I jumped without hesitation, almost missing the rock table below me. The murky water was carrying small logs and other debris that almost caught my feet. Had I been delayed a second or two the current could have swept me off my feet and carried me to a river. The water, however, just splashed on the solid base of my working tent. At least, the specimens we had collected during the last three weeks were safe. What luck!

Staying to the working tent to save the specimens would have been a terrible gamble. The site and sound of the rushing flood water made me leap instinctively!

The boys returned late that afternoon a little inebriated. They saw the havoc in our camp. The water system was destroyed. The split bamboos were scattered all over the campsite. Luckily our sleeping tents were far from the bank of the river. I cleaned the debris, but did nothing to fix the overall damage. We will do the mopping operation the next day. The boys became sober when they saw the mess. They thought I was angry. They had no idea about what had happened until I told them the story of the flash flood that thundered down towards our camp, carrying with it small logs and dead branches.

It was a terrifying experience to be alone in our camp.

I could only think of my "guide/guides" for making me jump at the right time!

17

A SIGN OF THE DEATH
OF MY FATHER

Mt. Isarog.was isolated, but we could communicate with my sister in Manila from the VHF (Very High Frequency) station. This VHF government transmitter was located at an altitude of 4,000 feet above sea level. It was an hour's climb from our camp through a rugged road designed for 4-wheel drive vehicles.

We made friends with the radio operators. One day, we received a direct message from the VHF that my father was very ill. He was on his last stage of cancer of the lungs. I decided to go home with my brother leaving my other younger brother with our two cousins. We missed the plane in Legaspi City so we took the night train to Manila where we could easily get a flight to my home province in Mindanao. The father of my cousins who was married to the younger sister of my mother, went with us. We took the night train that evening and arrived in Manila early the next morning. I went to my old boarding house where I usually left my personal belongings during long summer holidays.

My brother and the father of my cousins went out to buy some things that early evening. We were to fly to Mindanao early the next morning.

It was seven o'clock in the evening, on the 7th of May 1963. I was in my room. I flicked the switch on but the electric bulb would not light. Earlier, I had switched it on and it lit up. I went out to have dinner, switched it off, and came back. When I switched it on again it did not light. Maybe the life of the bulb has had it, I said to myself. Time to change the bulb, but I did not have any light bulb in the boarding house.

I remembered there was a candle somewhere in the room. This was a remembrance of my initiation to the Alpha Sigma Phi Fraternity. I found it and lighted it. The candle flame was so still. Usually a kind of flicker would show even without air current in the room. This was different. It was a continuous flow of bright light. It made me think my father must be breathing his last breath this very moment. May his soul rest in peace!

After about 20 minutes, the light bulb suddenly lighted up, as if somebody had switched it on. Who did it? This never happened in the two years I lodged in this place. It could have been a loose connection. Was it?

We took the plane to Cagayan de Oro City airport in Misamis Oriental and proceeded to my hometown by bus. When we arrived, my mother told me the exact time he passed away: seven o'clock in the evening. *That was the time I lighted a candle in my room in Manila. Was this a coincidence?*

Two days later, my father was buried in the Protestant cemetery in barrio Lunao, seven kilometers away from my hometown. His funeral brought together relatives from afar and all his friends. The cars and the throng of people that followed the cortege on foot extended for more than three kilometers. It was said that the line of mourners was the longest that attended a funeral in the history of the town. His grave was simple but it was full of the spirit and good wishes of people from different walks of life. Papa was a good man who helped others all the time. It was high time they gave respect to a person who had spent time rendering a little service to his fellowmen here and there—to anybody in dire need in our community. He was a Mason and a member of the local Lions Club.

I remember getting up suddenly after the minister's eulogy and recited by memory Psalm 23rd, 'The Lord is My Shepherd.' After all, I memorized this chapter when my father asked me to read the Book of Psalms seven years before his death. That was the time I courted death by somersaulting on the railing of the balcony on the second floor of Gingoog Institute and almost fell off to the concrete pavement 20 feet below. Understandably he was raging mad over the exhibitionist act I did.

As his casket was lowered to rest on the cold ground, I could not help but shed tears. He had worked all his life to support his family. I never told him I loved him, but I did love him, only I did not have the courage to tell him. He must know that I really loved him.

He wanted me to be a virtuous and honorable man.

I tried.

18

EXPOSURE TO MISSION WORK

After my third year of medical schooling, in 1964, the summer months of April and May led me to appreciate medical mission work. It was the beginning of a new pattern in my struggle for life and destiny. Evolving one step at a time, interconnected, yet unknown what the future would convey as the years passed, I realized then that the pattern had been set before me.

The mountain areas we explored were in Abatan, Buguias -- 90 kilometers north of Baguio City in the heart of northern Luzon.

We traversed a rough winding road following the ridge of a mountain range that led us to a mountain township. City dwellers at that time thought head hunting was still practiced in the hinterlands.

That thought occurred to me but only briefly as I decided that my expedition team should explore the central mountain areas of Luzon. I had thought of other areas, but to venture into this region without proper planning was a challenge. I studied the map of the area and traced with my finger the road from Baguio City to a place unknown to us -- the small town of Abatan, in the municipality of Buguias, in the province of Benguet. The fear of meeting head hunters was in our minds. We were all hesitant at first but the promise of a new adventure encouraged us brave and pure-hearted insect collectors to go ahead.

The party members were willing to go where I dared to go. The older brother of my cousin could not join us. Instead, a friend of my cousin, who was a taxi driver in Manila, was convinced of the thrills we would experience.

We took the Dangwa bus from Manila and another in Baguio City for Abatan.

We passed the highest mountain highway in the Philippines, and had lunch in a small restaurant in Sinipsip at 6,000 feet above sea level. It was windy and cold. It was 4°C at midday. We were half way to our destination. We thought that Abatan would have the same elevation as Sinipsip. It would be difficult and too cold to go out early in the morning to collect insect specimens. The bus started its gradual descent from Sinipsip to Abatan. We reached the place in mid-afternoon. The temperature was moderate.

At that time the population of Abatan was about 3,000. Most of the inhabitants were scattered in farm areas five to ten kilometers from the center of the small town. There were about 20 houses along the road and a couple of grocery stores. Abatan was situated in a crossroad that led to the Lepanto Mining Company in Mankayan and Buguias.

A medical clinic operated by the Lutheran Mission was approximately 60 meters away from where we temporarily rented a wooden house. The walls of the house were full of holes, and there were open spaces between the walls. It was cold! Nevertheless, we preferred being in this house rather than setting up our tents in the fields, where it would be much colder. The temperature was 6° C in the morning and 20°C at mid-day. This was supposed to be summer! In the cities the temperature would be between 35° and 40°C and very humid. The air here was fresh and it was foggy on most mornings. When we exhaled warm air from our lungs we can see steam coming out of our mouths.

The following day, I introduced the members of my collecting team and myself to the medical director, and his beautiful wife, Irene, who was one of the nurses. I told them that I was a medical student and would be in my fourth year come June.

I also met the American missionary pastor of the Lutheran church. He and his family and three children (Paula, Leah and Johnny) were staying at the Mission cottage which was properly insulated and warm. The well-built and insulated cottage was about 15 meters away from the clinic. Between the cottage and the clinic was a small Lutheran church with a large congregation. The Pastor had many converts after a few years of ministry.

The physicin-incharge and his wife were very accommodating. They introduced me to the few members of the staff: three nurses, three nursing aides, and a dietician. The clinic was open 24 hours a day. It admitted patients for a day or two, and provided intravenous fluids to patients who were severely dehydrated from gastroenteritis or in labor. Patients who needed major surgery or a complete work-up were sent to Baguio City or Manila. Patients with medical conditions like severe pneumonia, severe bronchitis or malaria, were admitted for a few days until they became well. Local midwives, who were employed by the government, referred difficult cases to the clinic.

After three days of collecting insects, I had the desire to help in the clinic. I asked the physician-in-charge of I could help around on certain days while my boys went about with

65

their usual chores. The physician was happy to have an assistant. I spent two or three hours in the afternoon helping the over-worked physician. He taught me many things as he treated different and difficult cases. This was where I learned to suture lacerations; do obstetrical deliveries, episiotomies and forceps deliveries. I was still a third year medical student. The textbook knowledge which I learned from the last semester was still very fresh in my mind. I applied my classroom and textbook knowledge as I helped the doctor treat cases.

What fascinated me for the first time was the case of a ten-year-old boy who had a three-inch laceration in his scalp after a motor vehicle accident. After the nurse had shaved the boy's hair, the physician said not to bother with local anesthesia.

"These people have a high threshold for pain."

I thought at first this was cruel to the child, suturing him with no anesthesia. The boy did not cry at all. Later, I learned that most of the patients tolerated stitching of wounds without local infiltration of procaine, the local anesthesia. I got used to it, while bearing the pain with them. The kids were not allowed by their parents to scream or cry. The father made them clench their teeth or bite a piece of cloth or wood. The kids diligently obeyed. (I compared this tribe to other tribes in the mountain areas and found that this Kankane-ey tribe in this locality had the highest threshold for pain). I wonder if this holds true now.

Sometimes, women in difficult labor for many hours strained in one corner of the clinic with their heads pressed against the wall. A friend, a neighbor or a nurse assisted them. Delivery sometimes took place in that nook. Frequently, when there was time, the woman walked to the delivery table in between contractions.

They had a special method of straining. The woman in labor would do a knee-chest position. As soon as she felt the baby's head was coming out she would lie down flat on her back on the concrete floor and give birth right then and there.

I was told that some husbands delivered their babies at home. They would call the rural health midwife when problems arose. If the government-trained midwife could not deliver the baby she would take the mother in labor to the clinic.

One case I could well recall. The mother was in difficult labor for more than 30 hours, was exhausted, and could hardly stand up when brought to the clinic. She had developed what we call in medical parlance uterine inertia (meaning the uterus is too weak to contract from exhaustion). The physician incorporated Pitocin in the intravenous drip and the woman delivered in just a few minutes. I simply assisted the delivery by catching the baby as it came out of the mother's private part. Three hours later, the intravenous fluids gave the woman new strength. The baby's umbilical cord was cut off, and in a couple of minutes the mother picked him up as if nothing had happened, and said she wanted to go home.

I asked her if she was strong enough (through an interpreter usually a nurse or a nursing aide).

The physician said, "That's common here."

Looking at the patient, a few feet away, the physician agreed, and let her go home. I could not forget this because the parents named their baby boy after me. I saw the birth certificate. Boy was I pleased.

The next few weeks, we moved our entomological camp to Lo-o valley, a few kilometers away, and in a much lower altitude. I divided my time between the clinic and field work. I hired an extra collector from the area who had befriended us to take over in my absence. I collected with them in the morning or arranged the specimens in pill boxes, layer by layer. In the afternoon and evenings, I spent my time in the clinic, and sometimes slept in one of the quarters. I became very interested in the medical and surgical cases.

One time, the physician asked me to take charge while he went to attend a medical conference in Manila. This was illegal practice of medicine, but this was better than having no student doctor at all. I survived without difficulty with the routine medical examinations. I had learned a bit of the local dialect, which was useful in asking medical questions and interviews.

Another day, I was alone. It was Sunday. The physician was in Baguio City attending another meeting sponsored by the Inter-Church Commission on Medical Care under the World Council of Churches. Baguio city was six to seven hours by car.

That afternoon, a bus fell off a ravine 15 meters deep, while on its way to the Lepanto Mining Company 20 kilometers away. Eight patients were brought to the clinic. Three had sustained severe multiple lacerations. There were no fractures though. I had to make a quick survey if somebody had internal damage. Luckily, there was none. It took me three hours to stitch all the lacerations. I was only a beginner but I managed. I thought that being new in the trade; it would take me a long time to learn to work on patients coming in. The nurses said, 'Doc, you did it quickly.'

After eight weeks in Abatan and the unexpected exposure to medical work in the mountains, we had to go back to Manila. I had good preparation for my fourth year in medical school.

The experiences I had that summer were gratifying but I wanted more. Five months later, in December 1964, I went back to the clinic. I had a ten-day Christmas break. I was seeking fulfillment that would reward a restless soul. Abatan was the place to find that. I was kept busy the seven days I was there. The physician and his wife had to take a few days off -- his Christmas break! He had complete trust in me. I saw many clinical cases quite different from those brought to the emergency room and Out- Patient Department of the UERMMC Medical Center.

In the outback, limited diagnostic facilities were a problem. The doctor had to depend most of the time on the patient's history, his hands, and clinical eyes. The gradual refinement of the doctor's clinical eye was far more important than ordering a series of laboratory procedures, X-rays, ultrasound, CT scanning. There was X-ray equipment in the Abatan Lutheran clinic. Ultrasound, CT., MRI was never heard of.

One time, we had a CPD (cephalo-pelvic disproportion) case, meaning the baby's head was too big for the pelvis of the mother. A *primigravida* (meaning first child), about four feet tall, was brought in. A small pregnant woman! You can imagine how small a four-foot tall woman is. She had active labor at home for more than 24 hours. After observing her for an hour with intravenous fluids running, we tried forceps. Pitocin drip was contra-indicated. Forceps failed, the baby's head was too big. We decided to transport the mother in the VW Kombi (converted to an ambulance) to Baguio City, on a precipitous winding road. At that time, the clinic had no equipment to perform an emergency C/S. Signs of fetal distress were positive. The night was very cold (it was the coldest time of the year). We had to hurry before the baby died inside the mother's womb. We were half of the way, when we noticed the mother was severely straining.

'It's coming out!' the small woman shouted in her local tongue.

We stopped immediately and took out the emergency delivery kit. I saw only the baby's head coming out of the mother's opening. Maybe the baby's shoulders were stuck. Finally, she gave a strong strain and the baby was out. The baby's head was very oblong. The head had molded itself against the small pelvic outlet. The baby gave a very faint cry. The light inside the van and the flashlight were not good enough to see the true color of the baby.

After a minute, the physician said, "The baby is very cyanotic," (meaning very dark blue). "Can you resuscitate?"

Without hesitation, in semi-lit condition, I did mouth- to- mouth resuscitation. There was a lot of mucus and meconium that I spat out. Soon after, the baby cried very softly, then louder. The baby's color changed. I felt relieved. By the time the baby was breathing spontaneously, the physician had extracted the placenta. I rushed out of the van. I vomited. The thought that I resuscitated the baby without wiping its mouth and face was nauseating. Several times, as we were going back to the clinic, the physician kept teasing me, asking how the meconium tasted.

"Revolting," I said.

Anyway, the next day, after a few hours of sleep, I could eat without getting nauseated, forgetting what happened the night before.

The event was all forgotten but the experience taught me always to clean well first the face especially the mouth area of the mother and the baby with gauze or something clean and dry.

There were many interesting tales about women unobtrusively delivering their babies.

For example, we heard that a woman had delivered her baby spontaneously in the field while harvesting potatoes. There was no word of labor difficulty or bleeding. She brought home her basket loaded with potatoes which she balanced on her head and a baby in her arms.

These women folk were physically tough in their daily living. They did not have any pre-prenatal check-up. Some did with the rural midwife. When a woman went out to till the soil or harvest crops, she walked up and down the hills with a baby wrapped in a blanket which was attached to her back.

The hard tasks that these inhabitants performed everyday produced in their system a natural pain killer. The brain can produce a morphine-line substance known as endorphin, which gives them strength.. This is probably the main reason delivery seemed so easy to most.

Forty years later today, the clinic is now the famous 50-bed Lutheran Hospital. It is well-equipped, catering to all sorts of emergencies and elective procedures. Surgeons are available at all times. In fact, my third child was delivered in this outback hospital.

19

A CRIPPLED ELDERLY

I was in my fourth year in medical school and had gained fair exposure to the medical world. The Out-Patient Department of UERM Memorial Center, the admitted cases, lectures, and clinico-pathological conferences were my greatest source of knowledge. The textbooks came second.

One afternoon, coming home from our regular classes, I noticed that an elderly woman, in her eighties, who lived across my boarding house, was in severe pain. She struggled to take a few steps near the doorway of her home. Her right knee was markedly swollen. I went and talked to her. I asked how she was with her condition and if the medication that she was taking was working or not.

"The medicines prescribed by the specialist are doing me no good," she said. "The weeks had been torture to me."

I asked myself why this elderly lady should suffer so much pain with all these modern pharmaceutical medicines in our midst. They work on some, but not on others. Maybe she needed an aspiration of the fluid in the knee or something else. Would they replace her knee at the stage of her life? (At that time knee replacement was not known.)

'I will touch your knee and when you wake up in the morning you will be able to walk again in comfort.' Without thinking, these words came out of my mouth, and jokingly, I touched her knee, but there was sincere kindness in my heart.

And she did! The next morning she walked over to my landlady and told her what had happened. I asked them not to tell anyone about what transpired especially the medical students and the interns. The information that "I was a faith healer" leaked out among a few houses in our street. I told them it was coincidence, and that the tablets that the specialist had given her had worked at the last minute.

I remembered the words written by one of America's pioneer physicians, Dr. Odler. These were written in the 19th century:

'It is not the doctor's prescription or diagnoses that is most important that heals, the mending bones that would knit by itself, or recovering from a severe infection, but it is one's faith that somehow the unexplainable happens from within the doctor's kindness and rapport.'

That old crippled lady must have felt the kindness in my heart. But to me there is something mystical about the woman's experience. Please read the pocket books like *Arigo the Surgeon with a Rusty Knife, Bruno Groening, Edgar Cayce,* etc.

20

INTERNSHIP: TWELVE MONTHS
OF GRINDING TASKS

This was the year I had to give up all extra-curricular activities. The fraternity had groomed me for the presidency of the Student Council that year (1966) but I turned it down. I felt that I needed more time to acquire more knowledge in medicine and clinical exposures. I was hungry for knowledge and thought of medical textbooks as irrelevant. I had gained medical knowledge mostly from lectures, clinico-pathological conferences, from bedside in-patients and from the out-patients and my experiences in the Abatan Lutheran Clinic.

The Internship year was a gruelling year in medical training. It was the grinding task in the physician's medical life.

Unlike in other rich countries, the interns in the Philippines are not paid for the services they perform. Interns have to pay for internship. The Philippines being a poor country, private medical schools and politicians want to put more money into their accounts. Indeed, to bear the strain of learning is affected heavily by one's financial condition.

My finances were at the lowest. I let my cousin, who was a Taxi driver in Manila, led a two-month expedition that summer in Montalban, near Manila. I saved a little money from that expedition without me leading the team. The money sent by Bishop Museum in Hawaii was cut by 50 per cent. My sister who was a journalist helped me through the year. I could not make any gains for an entomological expedition as there was no time. After the fourth year term ended we took a few days off then returned to school promptly to commence 12 months of internship.

Recalling the Internship year, it was the hardest yet the happiest year of all, not only for me, but for others too. Maybe there were a few who did not find it so hard. It was the year the physicians could appreciate Shakespeare's words: 'Those who have not experienced the worst of life's bitters can never appreciate the sweetest of things.'

Indeed, the contentment, and the inner satisfaction one feels are aptly defined by John Ruskin: 'The highest reward for a man's toil is not what he gets for it but what he becomes by it.'

The 24-hour duties and the sleepless nights, all these I can remember well. Twenty four hours of duty, two or three times a week, followed by the normal working hours during the day -- a total of 32 hours without a wink could really test one's endurance. During those times, when one was on duty, no one could take a brief nap. It was not allowed. Another 24-hours duty was imposed if one was caught taking a nap.

One intern was caught taking a nap. He was assigned another 24 hours at the Emergency Room or the Casualty Section. The Chief Resident (Senior Resident) on duty was there all the time checking where the intern was. When paged and no answer was received he had to give a valid reason.

The grinding year could break one's mind. I remember a classmate who assisted a major operation after a 24-hour duty in the wards. He slumped on the patient while on sterile drapes. He was punished for not being able to keep himself awake! Was that cruel? So, he had to work in the Emergency Room for other 24-hours of duty. The third day, he had to assist another elective operation. He became pale and sweaty but he held on. The weekend saved him and he got his long lost sleep.

When a similar incident happened to another Intern, he broke down, and could not finish Internship.

Luckily I did not get any punishment.

One can imagine one's jitters and anxiety after a sleepless night. This was expressed in the Intern's face especially when the Consultant was a "terror." One morning a lady intern in my group (of five) was asked by this particular "terror" Consultant to examine the patient again and to listen to her heart murmur.

'How can you appreciate the heart sounds when your stethoscope is not in your ears?' The Consultant, with a raised voice, probably laughed to himself afterward.

The daily struggles and difficulties of Internship came to pass. We felt gratified for it had prepared us for the future. When grim obstacles confronted us in actual practice in future years, we were prepared to maintain ourselves with forbearance and a clear mind. This was the ultimate lesson we learned in our own experience. This setting molded our minds and spirits.

We perceived a feeling of inner contentment that filled our hearts with the molding ordeals. They made us appreciate that somehow gentleness existed in real life aside from the pain and suffering we saw most often. It was in this perspective that we saw our desires, staying ever hopeful, though one's world might have been turbulent.

One memorable experience I cherished was when we were interns for three months in another hospital—Labor Hospital, Project 4, Quezon City, now known as the Quirino Memorial Hospital. At that time it was known as Labor Hospital which catered only to maternity cases.

I did not mean to break any existing record. This happened spontaneously. One counted the number of obstetrical deliveries done in 24 hours. I broke the record by delivering 17 neonates in 24 hours. It was that particular October in 1965. This month is the peak month for deliveries in most hospitals

The day started at eight o'clock in the morning. My third delivery at nearly ten o'clock was relatively an easy one. After a couple of hours of labor, this multipara (meaning she had delivered many, six actually in this case) made a strong and continuous strain for approximately 10 seconds. The baby emerged from the mother's womb with very minimal discomfort. After the placenta was extracted, Ergotrate was routinely administered intramuscularly to prevent the uterus from relaxing, thus preventing hemorrhage. A few minutes later, the woman was wheeled hurriedly to her bed in her assigned ward.

There was another woman who was in brisk labor in the hallway. The cervix was fully effaced, ready to deliver any minute. There were two obstetrical tables in the delivery room, one for my partner, the other for me. Most of the time we delivered the babies ourselves with no senior resident close by as he may be occupied somewhere else. He is paged only when obstetrical problems arise. Most of the women who came in for delivery had no pre-natal check up. They showed up at the hospital when they were already in active uterine contractions.

It was past 12 o'clock, mid-day. I had already delivered four babies routinely without complications. There was no Pediatric Intern to help resuscitate newborns. If there was resuscitation to be done we had to do it ourselves. The bell or a buzzer was put through to the Nurse Station for the Chief Senior Resident to come if we thought something dreadful was imminent.

It was noon-break. As I passed by the bed of my third case, I accidentally glimpsed at her. I noticed her to be pale and somewhat in distress. Patients could not complain because they knew everybody was busy. I went to her and asked if she was all right.

'I have pains in the pit of my stomach,' she answered.

I felt for her uterus and found this was way up in the epigastrium or pit of the stomach. I rushed to the Chief Senior Resident who was on his way to the dining room. I told him I suspected something was wrong with the patient. There was a possibility of a ruptured lower uterine segment as the contracted uterus was way up high in the epigastrium or stomach area. The Chief Resident asked me a brief resume of the delivery. I told him it was normal except that after the placenta was extracted there was very minimal bleeding.

'Go back and catheterize her.' His face showed no concern.

I knew he was hungry as I was. I was desperate. I knew something was wrong with the patient, but he would not come with me. I went to catheterize the woman and took the vital signs. She was irritated by this procedure and I ran back quickly to the Chief Resident.

"Sir, please see this patient. No urine came out. Her BP is 80/60 mm Hg. The pulse is faint and thread. She is very pale." I was almost jumping, not in excitement, but in fear of the patient's life that was in danger.

The Resident Doctor went and had a quick look and his clinical eyes had the impression of a massive hemorrhage. He ordered the nurse to rush the patient to the Emergency Operating Table while paging for the OR nurses to come urgently.

"STAT!" That was the code word.

The patient was wheeled into the OR (short for operating room) immediately. An 18-gauge needle was inserted right away by the Chief Resident in the cubital fossa. Luckily he found one and a plasma expander was pumped right away, while he was raising his voice ordering Type O blood (no cross-matching, mind you). "Order three liters."

"Shout at everybody to run!"

He quickly infiltrated the lower abdominal wall with 20 to 30 cc of local anesthetic. He grabbed a scalpel, after putting on his surgical globes without scrubbing. The patient was in circulatory shock, pale and semi-conscious, gasping for air even with the oxygen mask on.

He cut the abdomen with a few strokes below the navel and dark blood poured out of the abdominal cavity. The nurse who was manning the suction could hardly cope with the flood of bright red blood in the open abdomen. In one minute or even less from the time he cut the abdominal wall, his left hand was blindly directing the long curved forceps to the spurting uterine artery of the ruptured lower uterus. I could see the flow of bright red blood mixing with the dark venous blood. The bleeder was still there!

"The uterine artery is difficult to feel, he said excitedly. "Hand me a clamp," he commanded. "Another clamp." "Another clamp, please. Thanks."

A few seconds passed and the stream of bright red blood stopped.

"We got the bleeder," the Senior Resident said calmly now after taking a pause and heaving a deep sigh of relief. He then removed his gloves, scrubbed his hands, and finished the operation the aseptic way.

The left uterine artery was severed with the rupture of the left lower uterine segment. This probably happened as the woman made the last forceful strain in the Delivery Room. A total hysterectomy was done without the consent of the patient or relatives.

This patient could have died in her bed from massive internal hemorrhage with only a few minutes delay while in her bed. I would have been in hot water. Would I?

What made me look at her? There was an intuitive feeling that something was wrong. This is where the clinical eyes are trained. *But what made me look at her when I was rushing to the dining room for lunch? Was this luck or "guidance" from the mystical world?*

The following week, we had a clinico-pathological conference of this episode. I presented the case of the woman who nearly died. I remember, my Co-Intern, my best friend at that time, now a practicing psychiatrist in US saying, "You could have been given an award, even a congratulatory word for having picked up the case with your eyes."

The honor went to the Chief Resident who acted as the emergency surgeon who really saved the patient's life. There was no appreciation given for what I had done. It did not matter. What mattered was the patient lived to tell the tale and she said when she was discharged that she was more grateful to me than to anybody else.

I still had 18 more hours of duty.

Lionel was on the "losing end." The cases I admitted were delivered quicker than his. When there was an emergency admission (as usual they were in active labor) the admitting nurse would ring the bell. I would tell Lionel to go and see the new admission because my patient's cervix was fully dilated and any time she could deliver. I assured him that I would look after his case in the next delivery table. He accepted hesitantly. By the time he came back, I had delivered his case that he had been attending to for over an hour. This continued throughout the night and a few times I delivered his case. By eight o'clock in the morning, I had delivered 17 babies into the world.

This was halfway through our internship. And there was still a lot more to learn.

Internship was an immense experience. We saw the struggle between life and death. We heard the desperate cries of women in labor, and the screams of relatives of patients who died. We heard the loud cry of a newborn baby. An old man's dying wish. We saw and smelled the filth and dirt in our ward, and we had to practice tidiness and cleanliness, we had to be conscious of many things.

One intriguing fact circulating among the interns was that one Senior Resident was called "Jinx!" Whenever this SMR was on duty for 24 hours, the hospital Emergency Room and the wards were very busy with very serious patients dying all through the night. When another Senior Surgical Resident was on duty the whole hospital seemed quiet. Some interns felt this too. When Dr. J. C. was on, everything happened. Dr. C. is now medical director of St. Luke's Global Medical Center, one of the country's best modern hospitals.

I got very busy too most days but not one died in my hands. Dr. Lionel said he signed 17 death certificates in 12 months. This number was the number of babies I delivered a few months earlier in another hospital. Was it luck? I did not sign any death certificate throughout my 12 months of Internship.

One time, we had a post-craniotomy case. A brain tumor was removed. Lionel and I alternated taking care of this patient every other day. Every time Lionel was on call the vital signs fell. When it was my turn, the vital signs stabilized.

The following days, that room where the patient died, was haunted. The room number was 13 on the fourth floor. Nurses observed that something happened in that suite in the middle of the night even if there was no patient inside. Some patients claimed they saw somebody in white attire walking about, but nobody entered that room that night. Was there a ghost? I wonder if some hospital had these things going on! A lot believe in the supernatural. Do you?

The last days culminated with a comprehensive examination. If one did not pass this, he had to repeat internship. Of the 100 interns, only one had to repeat the course again. There were 301 of us when we were enrolled the first year.

After 12 months of hard work as an intern, I felt a change in me. I felt sad, yet there was inner serenity that filled my heart. At last I have not failed Internship. I made it despite my financial difficulties!

When we left the hospital grounds of the medical school, 12 months of hardship seemed so short. Our deeds and struggles were embedded in our memory once our hearts got lost. Now we understood. The sweet confusion made us perceive a new horizon of uncertainties.

We became insignificant again.

21

THE LAST EXPEDITIONARY FLING

After taking the medical board examination, we had four months of waiting for the results. The results were to be published in the newspapers. I did not go out with the new doctors and have fun to compensate for the gruelling exams.

Instead, I spent my last fling at an entomological expedition. I wrote Dr. Quate if Bishop Museum would sponsor an expedition I would organize; fortunately, the answer was in the affirmative. We would be collecting bugs and insects in deeper territories of northern Luzon. Funds were provided.

This time we went to Mayoyao, Ifugao, in the heart of northern Luzon. We made a quick stop at Abatan to greet old friends, and then proceeded to Banaue via Bontoc and to our new destination, Mayoyao. The provincial road ended in this town. The town of Mayoyao was 42 kilometers east of Banaue. The famous rice terraces of Banaue attracted foreign and Manila-based tourists. The terraces in Mayoyao area were far more beautiful than those of Banaue, but few tourists could visit the Mayoyao terraces because of the inaccessibility of land transportation.

I was glad when I found out there was a 12-bed Mission Hospital in Mayoyao. I could help the doctor assigned there during my spare time. The hospital ground was located on top of a mountain, overlooking the town, 500 meters below us. It was an ideal place to spend the holidays in.

There were 17 villages in the district of Mayoyao. They loomed at a distance along rice terraces. In a downward slope, some sitios or barangays were 10 to 30 kilometers away from the town proper. The farthest was Bunhian, 30 kilometers away. This was situated east of the town near the Isabela border (Isabela is the province east of Ifugao).

The miniature hospital was originally built by the Philippine Jaycees in the 1950s and was later endorsed to the United Church of Christ in the Philippines in the 1960s.

We established our camp about 50 meters away and above the hospital grounds. This was on an elevated area overlooking the well-irrigated green rice terraces. We could tell that harvest time was near as the rice plantations looked verdant.

We made friends with physician-incharge and his family. They did not have kids. The few members of the staff were "locals" from the community. Some of the personnel had obtained their education in Baguio City or Manila.

At first the local inhabitants eyed us suspiciously; we noticed this the first week we went out to collect specimens around the sides of the mountain. We had to walk through the grand rice terraces to get into the forest.

Somebody started a damaging rumor that we went to the source of the town's water supply and put poison in their drinking water. This spread like wildfire. They thought we were communists. Communists were everywhere in the Philippines at that time – whether in Manila or the provinces.

Then one day, a group gathered around our camp with their dubious posture, holding their native spears. We had made friends with a few but still a lot were unfriendly. In fact, we hired one local inhabitant to be a member of our team. Others were not convinced that we were only collecting insects in the vicinity. They claimed we had some "fishy reason" behind this expedition. It was a good thing the local chief executive, the Mayor, dispelled this idea and told his constituents that we were insect collectors for a museum in the US and that I had just finished my medical schooling in Manila. And that we were not "communists."

The ancestors of these natives used to be head-hunters, and some of their descendants still carry the tradition of severing the heads of their enemies. In fact, two years before we arrived in the area, the hospital staff told us, a Caucasian missionary priest was beheaded. I was friendly with the townsfolk, believing that making friends was better than using guns or force. Before I knew it, everybody was good to me and my team.

One day, the municipal treasurer of the town visited me in my working tent. He told me about a medical problem that had been bothering him for more than six months. He was really worried. He was told he had a heart problem and that the chest pains he had was angina. I listened to his medical history and examined him quickly. If he had a heart problem he would not be able to walk up to my tent from the town. That was more than a stress test.

I told him that it was reflux esophagitis or heartburn. I told him to get antacids and to refrain from drinking whisky, coke, coffee, and eating spicy food. A few days later, he came back to our camp, declaring happily that he did not have chest pains anymore. Grateful for what I had done, he recommended me to his friends who had lingering medical problems. The physician running the small hospital must have heard of my seeing a few patients for free in my working tent. He was not pleased, I assumed.

He resigned and moved out in a few days. To me, I was not the main reason why he resigned. It was an opportunity for him to leave. Almost all the doctors assigned to this most isolated place could not stay more than six months. They found excuses so that they could leave the place. Meanwhile, the local treasurer communicated with the main office of the UCCP in Quezon City, endorsing me to take over. I was not licensed yet to practice medicine. I was not sure if I had passed the board exams. I had a few months to wait for the result.

Seeing the pain and suffering of the sick natives touched my heart. So, I accepted the offer after our entomological work was over. I took the chance of working in that mission hospital for two months without a license. I told the church representative I would not be responsible if something dreadful happened. The UCCP main office agreed to put me on board anyway.

My expeditionary team had ended two months of delightful work. They all went back to Manila except my brother, Lemuel, who stayed with me for a few more weeks.

One afternoon, I tasted the local brewed rice wine with a few friends in the small town. The Mayor came out and congratulated me for having passed the board exams. I was surprised. The paper he read was a week old. My best friend in medical school forgot to send me a telegram that I had passed; I was waiting for that. I had two days to go to catch the oath-taking ceremony in Manila. It took me 30 hours to reach Manila by bus.

I took my Hippocratic Oath on time.

That was the last time I saw the faces of my classmates. They had struggled with me for five years in the pursuit of medical knowledge. The gruelling medical training at that time was excellent. We could now face partly the sick world on our own with confidence.

The next step for us was to go into specialization. Most of my classmates who went to the United States became specialists in their chosen fields. Not me. I was stuck in the hinterlands.

22

DREAMS SHATTERED: I DRIFTED INTO THE UNKNOWN FUTURE

I accepted the position in Mayoyao Mission Hospital after passing the board exams. My dream of becoming a trained surgeon was placed on hold. Was it meant to be? I was in a place so remote from civilization only a few doctors who were assigned there in the past could endure the hardship for a few months.

I promised myself I would stay only for a year then hopefully find my way to one of the large training hospitals in the U.S. I had earlier applied for surgical residency in Flower Hospital, Ohio, after my internship. I received a letter from the hospital that I was accepted. However, I could not go that year. I was working in the hinterlands of Luzon, in a place that my college professor would have called "God-forsaken country."

I was the lone physician available to attend to the medical needs of a population of 17,000 at that time. The local inhabitants were scattered in many villages. Patients came from these villages as far as 20 kilometers away for consultation, confinement or surgery -- by foot, or, for non-ambulatory cases, carried in a rattan hammock. I felt like "Tom Dooley" in the area.

The first two months kept me real busy. The locals tested me for their chronic and acute medical conditions. There were severe cases of anemia from chronic malaria, acute cases of malignant malaria, tuberculosis, and other infectious diseases which had not been treated properly. Many could not comply with the required long-term therapy due to lack of funds. A lot of them earned their income from the produce of their rice terraces. This was not enough for their own needs for the whole year. Very few could sell their harvest and earn extra cash for medical expenses. Some depended on relatives working in the cities for financial help.

There were dramatic acute conditions that were treated in a short time. Major surgical cases were referred to a general hospital in Banaue. Traveling to that place at that time, by a four-wheeled vehicle (converted to ambulance) took at least four hours (42 kilometers) of breath-taking ride on a one-- lane narrow road. Most parts of the road were carved from the granite walls of the mountains. I was told this was done early in the 1930s when the Americans used dynamite to blast the granite rocks. On the right or left side of the road was a sheer vertical drop 500 or 1000 feet below.

One day, in early 1967, the area was terribly affected by a strong typhoon. This hit northern Luzon. A day after the typhoon, the region was shaken by an earthquake of moderate intensity. It moved a mountain, and a stretch of road, two hundred meters long, vanished. Our link with civilization was cut off. The only means of locomotion was by foot. The road that vanished was on a sheer steep side of a mountain. To build a new road around the mountain would be more expensive for the government. This could take a long time. The repair was done by hand. Bulldozers intended to work in the area could not come as they were clearing landslides in many other places during the next two months.

I knew I would face a dilemma sooner or later. I could not refer surgical cases. No helicopter or transport for serious or surgical cases was available. (The American Subic Base was one that could render such service, but when I was in Mayoyao, no case was transported by a U.S. helicopter.) The only telephone in the area located was cut off in many places. Banaue, 42 kilometers far from Mayoyao, had a landing strip for small planes which ferried very serious cases to Baguio or Manila.

The inevitable came! A female patient had been transported by jungle hammock from her village ten kilometers away. She had lost a lot of blood. I was frantic, looking for blood donors. I did the blood typing and the cross-matching as the miniature hospital had no laboratory technician. There was nobody that matched her blood group except mine. She was lucky. I extracted 350 cc of my blood from my veins using the 500 cc citrated bottle.

I had to "go in" urgently before she would bleed again. We did an emergency Classical Caesarean Section under local anesthesia with only a nurse assisting. I made it. The first major operation I did on my own. Somehow my hands did not shake; nor did I have slight tremors. The operation seemed easy! I was elated that I could do it. Her recovery was uneventful.

The next day, I had a case of acute appendicitis. I had to "open up" the patient before the appendix ruptured and caused peritonitis, a deadly complication. I did a low-spinal anesthesia using a hyperbaric solution. This prevented the escape of the spinal anesthesia up the upper spine which may cause death.

The appendix was gangrenous and markedly swollen, ready to burst at the slightest pressure. I was able to take this out slowly without spillage.

The problem arose when I tried to close the abdominal wall. The guts were popping out caused by the increased intra-abdominal pressure. The patient was half-awake and she would strain when I tried to close the abdomen. The level of anesthesia was up to the navel only. I could not get a good relaxation of her abdominal muscles. I ordered more Valium and Demerol. Still the small intestine slipped out and I could not push it back inside. When I pushed a segment of the gut, another segment of the small intestine would slide through the incision. It seemed there was a lot of gas building up in the intestine.

'My God, there is plenty of gas inside the gut! How can I close this?' I was inaudibly talking to myself. I could feel the sweat in my forehead and under my surgical gown.

The nurse who assisted me read my mind as I placed my hands over a large sponge shoving the intestine in. She knew I was in a fix. As the patient was partially sedated, she strained whenever I shoved in the slippery gut. More of the small intestine came out so I had to put it back with my two hands preventing all the guts to spill out of the entire abdominal cavity. I could not ask the nurse what the other doctors did before when things like this happened

I felt my heart racing! She had enough Demerol and Valium intramuscularly yet she was still resisting

"Look for Prostigmin!" I ordered this drug. I had hoped this would not rupture the stump were the appendix was taken out. The nurse aide could not find the Prostigmin. I begged her to keep looking. Finally, she found the only Prostigmin ampoule. This was slowly given intravenously. The guts went inside the abdominal cavity with a gentle shoving of my hands. What a relief! The closure layer by layer was easily done. Nobody knew that I was perspiring under the surgical gown and had a chill, bone deep, and fine tremor in my whole body.

The next four weeks, surgical cases seemed to come up every day. What kind of training was I getting? I was training myself and applying a lot of what I learned from my internship. There were miscarriages, difficult forceps deliveries, strangulated hernias, an ectopic pregnancy, a hacked arm with a severed brachial artery. There were other medical conditions such as tuberculosis, pneumonia, amebiasis, malaria, and a lot more. Bless my soul! Angel luck was with me. At least I did not have any mortality.

The road was finally opened after two months. The means of transport were restored. There was a minibus three days a week. Our converted ambulance (a 4-wheel drive jeep), the Mayor's jeep, the four-wheel-drive vehicle that was operated by the Catholic School below the town, and my Trail Honda motorcycle were the only modes of transport in the whole community.

By then, I had developed confidence in so short a time doing surgical explorations mostly under spinal or local anesthesia. We did not have to refer most surgical cases. Luckily, the hyperbaric spinal anesthesia did not give me any complications.

Was there a mystical protection?

23

MY MAYOYAO EXPERIENCE

I was 29 years of age when I had a very strange experience in Mayoyao. This happened in March 1967.

WILL IT EVER COME BACK?

I glanced at the clock on top of a rattan-made shelf at the side of my bed when I was awakened by something I did not know. It was exactly three o'clock in the morning. All of a sudden a sense of well-being came to me and I was fully awake. I changed into my casual clothes, went out of my quarters, started my motorcycle and took off without telling the nurse on duty where I was going. She must have been surprised that I left without letting her know. It was crazy of me not to tell her. (At that time, I was the lone physician in Mayoyao, a far-flung area. I ran a 12-bed community hospital, and my sleeping quarter was only 15 meters away.)

From the hospital premises, on top of the levelled mountain, I rode down to the town, on a winding road. Then proceeded further, two kilometers down, where the United Church of Christ in the Philippines chapel made of wood was situated. I parked my motorcycle on a plain playground 50 meters away from the chapel.

Why did I come here? Was I dreaming, motor cycling in my sleep? At 3 o'clock in the morning? I tried to wake myself. I pinched strongly my skin. I was awake!

It was totally dark when I switched off the motorcycle engine and the sky was moonless though starlit. I wondered if somebody heard the sounds of the motorcycle. There were houses nearby. They must have thought I was out of my mind to be riding out here in this unholy hour. They knew I was the only one who had the motorcycle in the community. It seemed though that all the townsfolk were deep in their slumber. Not a soul in view, not a sound could be heard. It felt eerie.

Something in my mind was initiating, trying to pour out words as if it wanted me to make an extemporaneous speech. What for? Did somebody possess me? Suddenly, words from my mouth thundered out but it was clearly my voice. I spoke words spontaneously as though knowledge of many things had been stored in my brain for ages and were now coming out— some knowledge I'd not known before. The sentences I uttered were perfectly systematized and organized without pre-meditation or speculation. I was orating extemporaneously!

It was a tremendously great feeling!

The stream of thoughts, pouring out perfectly from my tongue was incredible. That episode lasted 15 minutes or a little more, loud and clear without hesitation. Then I stopped, and asked myself, where did I get all this information? How is it possible that I could be preaching now, and never before? My memory was not that good to retain such knowledge yet at this very instant I was overwhelmed with inexhaustible knowledge!

I started back to the hospital, still in total darkness, gripped with fear by what happened but still wished that the state of mind I had possessed would remain. If this state would stay forever, I even thought of becoming a great politician and possibly become one day The President of the Philippines.

I must have been away from the hospital for almost an hour. As I rode back up to the hospital about a thousand feet elevation from where I was, I sensed I was going back to my old self again. I felt the euphoric feeling draining away.

I could not tell the nurse on duty where I went. I went back to bed but could not sleep anymore. I was my real self again and I asked myself:

"Did I do sleep walking?" It could not be because every second that I did, I fully remembered.

"Or was I possessed by a Spirit?" If I was, I would have not remembered every minute of what happened.

"Or was it due to something I must have eaten before I went to bed." I tried to remember what I ate that night. Nothing was unusual.

Or did I happen to take a tablet? I did not take any kind of tablet or any drug by hand,

The nurse on duty, asked me where I went at that unholy hour. I told her, I could not sleep so I took a "stroll" with my Honda motorcycle.

This beautiful but strange experience lingered on for months, which I never told anybody. Nonetheless, I was longing for more.

Forty seven years had passed, but that experience never came back.

I asked Mrs. Pam P., years later when I was in Sydney, the clairvoyant I admired if I was possessed by a spirit and she said, "Elijah!"

If one has read the book ***Arigo: Surgeon of the Rusty Knife*** written by John Grant Fuller, one will surely know what possession by a spirit is all about. But "possession of a good Spirit" is an extremely rare phenomenon in human history.

In a particular case, Arigo, who was only a coal miner in Brazil in the early 1950s, became possessed by the spirit of a Portuguese physician whenever he prayed "The Lord's Prayer." He could then cure a dreadful malady or a far-advanced cancer with a rusty kitchen knife. At the time of his possession he did not have any consciousness of what had happened, only to realize, when he awakened, that he had cured people. Arigo did not charge any fee at all for he believed that the gift given to him was not to be used for enriching himself.

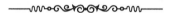

In my case, what happened in 1967 when I was possessed by a spirit for about 15 minutes? I was conscious all the time.

24

THE SECOND TIME I GAVE MY OWN BLOOD

One surgical procedure I performed was emergency exploratory laparotomy on a patient who had an acute abdomen problem. This always remained fresh in my memory.

When I operated on a young small woman, 18 years of age, under spinal anesthesia, it turned out she had an abdominal pregnancy. She was single and the thought of ectopic pregnancy did not enter my mind. Ultrasound, CT or MRI were not known at the time.

As I explored the lower abdomen cavity, I felt with my forefinger (of course with sterile gloves on) that I punctured something soft and spongy. It was the placenta adhering to the back of the abdomen between the right kidney and the urinary bladder. With only one nurse assisting, I suctioned the remaining blood to clear the operating field with a simple 100 cc irrigation syringe. Then we cleared a large amount of dark blood by displacing the gut with large gauze and retractors.

The placenta was clearly shown. It was the size of a small saucer, about four to five inches in diameter. The spot where I probed my finger was oozing with fresh blood. This was an abdominal pregnancy. Where was the bleeding coming from before I punctured the placenta? Where was the fetus? Maybe it came with the clots of blood that I took out manually. I found the right fallopian tube markedly enlarged. This had ruptured, and bleeding came from that portion. The fetus must have been enlarging at the distal end of the fallopian tube but the placenta grew in the abdominal wall. I could not believe that I would encounter a situation such as this. I did. This was a very rare happening even in big hospitals. The fetus could not be found. If the fetus was outside the fallopian tube, it could have survived and even attain the normal gestation process. This is termed peritoneal pregnancy.

Blood was rapidly oozing fast from where I punctured the placenta! My God, how can I stop the bleeding? There was no instrument to extricate this adherent placenta. I started to panic!

My God, please help me! I could not utter this in front of my only assistant, a nurse, and to the circulating nursing aide. Both of them were trained in the OT (Operating Table). If I remove my surgical gloves and looked for donors there would be a slim change I could find one. I went around the clinic, looking for blood donors. By the time I had cross-matched a few, the patient would probably be in circulatory shock.

'Use the best instrument in the world!' This thought came to my mind.

There was very little time to pause and meditate. I dug and scraped the placenta with my fingers. I felt the soft, tender pliable tissues easily breaking up. Later, I scraped the remaining small fragments of the placenta with strips of gauze.

Her vital signs went down.

'Pump more saline,' I ordered. We had run out of plasma expander. After a while it was all clear, every bit of placental tissue was extricated.

The whole ordeal took almost one and a half hours, my neck was stiff, and my knees were shaky.

Boy was I exhausted!

My problem was not over yet. The patient needed blood. I had to do blood typing of the few relatives who were around. None would match from among those who wanted to donate blood. There were two friends who matched with her blood type but were too scared to give blood. My blood matched with her. I extracted 350 cc of blood from my own vein. This was my second time to donate blood to a patient I operated on.

It felt good to give new life. My blood ran into the patient's system. Post-operatively, some blood was draining into the drainage bottle connected to the side of the abdominal wall!

'My God, she is still bleeding from somewhere! Please Lord, let her live. Should she die this can cost me my scalp!' One can not underestimate the temperament of the native tribe. How can I prepare their minds to accept the inevitable?

The night was restless, the hours seemed long. I kept waking up and checking her condition.

Morning came. She wanted to eat. The drain was no longer oozing blood and bowel sounds were present. That was quick! The bowel sounds were music to my ears.

The blood I freely gave so that I might save a life.

And I did.

25

THE UNKNOWN PREPARATION

After several months of mission work, life continued to be thrilling and exciting. There was no mortality among my surgical cases. If there were deaths, they were medical conditions beyond my control like far-advanced tuberculosis, pneumonia, cerebral malaria, severe malnutrition and other infectious diseases. Other doctors who had been in Mayoyao before could only stay a few months, discouraged by the terrible primitive conditions. I lasted much longer than any doctor before. It must have been a God-forsaken place in the consciousness of others but for me—it was dreamland.

Mayoyao must be different now 47 years after I left the place. I heard a government hospital was built in the *poblacion*. There were two doctors employed by the government and they were residents of the locality. The small hospital I used to spend some time had been closed but the buildings are still there. The instruments have been pilfered.

I was turning 29 years of age and my application for residency at Flower Hospital in Ohio, U.S.A. was accepted. My plans to go abroad had long been shelved. I had four months to go to serve the Mayoyao community and I was not renewing my contract.

Medical mission work was my craving and to serve the needy gave me an inner satisfaction, of well-being. I felt pain for those afflicted when the hospital budget was cut. It was sad seeing patients dressed in their usual G-strings squeeze out from their woven native-made wallet their last peso bill so they could pay their medical bill. Patients sometimes paid in kind: a chicken, a piglet, a cow for major operations. I accepted the payments in kind. I raised the poultry. I built pig pens, and had two cows mowing in the lower grounds behind my quarters.

We could not afford to give people too much charity. People abused this and we felt it. This is the reason the church cut the budget. Everything was not meant to be free.

Nevertheless, unknown events started to interfere with my dream for the future. I was meant to meet my destiny. One day, I attended a conference in Manila. When I returned from Manila via Bontoc, a pharmaceutical sales representative introduced me to a pretty new graduate who was helping out at the Bontoc Provincial Hospital. She was waiting for her nursing board exam result. I told her we needed another nurse in the hospital in Mayoyao and if she could work in our place that would be great!

When I met Nellie the second time, my heart and soul fell for her. Cupid's dart had pierced my heart.

We got married after three months in her hometown, Sagada, Bontoc, 120 kilometers away from Mayoyao. It was one of the biggest wedding celebrations in the town. The whole community was there and some folks from neigh- boring town of Besao were there too. There were a total of at least 5,000 guests, I was told. I realized then that the poultry, pigs, and cows I was intending to sell for my ticket to the United States turned out to feed a multitude in Sagada during our wedding day. I had that feeling afterwards that I had unknowingly raised all those animals in preparation for my wedding day. I was glad I had those animals waiting and ready to be served on my wedding day!

We went to Baguio City and planned to proceed to Manila for our honeymoon for two weeks. However, while we were in Baguio City on our second day of honeymoon, we received a telegram from the hospital administrator begging us to go back as there were emergency cases. They did not want to be referred to other hospitals.

Back to work again!

To me, it was a great pleasure returning to my task. The interruption of our honeymoon did not matter much. I adored the environment and the place was excellent and romantic for a honeymoon the whole year round. The beauty of nature can be appreciated from the hospital ground, near and far. The Philippine Jaycees built this 12-bed hospital complete with surgical and dental instruments. It was built on a levelled mountaintop flattened by manual labor. The location was 500 meters above the town proper.

The townsfolk called it "the hospital above the clouds" for good reason. Some days when there were signs of impending rain, the hospital looked like it was sitting on clouds.

The hospital had room for 12 beds, yet during epidemics it could accommodate 30 patients. Patients slept on the hallway. Sometimes some slept on locally- made mats on the floor.

My wife and I decided to stay a few more months in Mayoyao. I had been there for 18 months already. According to my friend, the mayor of Mayoyao, I was the only physician who had stayed the longest in the place. The hospital board looked for a replacement. My plan for further specialization abroad did not materialize. Still there was a glimmer of hope in my heart about going to the US someday.

Deep in my heart I found solace in the jungles. I really did not want to leave the place as I felt for the people and I had satisfaction in my sacrifice. However, changes happened beyond my dreams and expectations. I began to think of the future for my family and me? Would I be staying in Mayoyao forever? My wife was already pregnant with our first child. I asked myself and my mind found the answer… 'To accept things I cannot change.'

Before my term ended, I was offered a challenging position as Medical Director and Administrator of St. Theodore Hospital in Sagada, Bontoc Province. This was a 45-bed hospital with its seven out-station Clinics. The clinics were manned by nurses. They were located in different mountain provinces. After careful study, I accepted the offer. There were two doctors in the hospital. I did not have to be on call seven days a week. This was great!

It was another challenge I met with delight. In another four months, in April 1968, I would be in another mission.

I worked at St. Theodore Hospital for only a year on account of internal problems incurred by the previous administrators. I decided to move on, wanting to work in a more peaceful environment.

26

WHEN IT WAS TIME TO LEAVE, IT WAS TIME TO LEAVE!

I t is always difficult leaving a place you have grown to love. Departure day in Mayoyao was full of sadness. We had gotten accustomed to the place and made new friends there. Eighteen months seemed so short.

In some way, the restless spirit within me wanted more experiences. I was always optimistic that the future would bring something new, something different. I was hoping the new assignment will not result in failure. But we had to look for other frontiers.

In May 1969, my wife and I moved to Dagupan, Tabuk, Kalinga-Apayao to establish our own private clinic

Tabuk is in the central plains, in the heart of northern Luzon. Opened after World War II, it was considered a rich town and the rice granary of northern Luzon. People from different parts of the country migrated to this town. The place recorded the highest temperature in the country at 44°C at that time. During summer the sweltering heat was unbearable without an electric fan or an air-conditioning unit. We could not afford any of these yet. There was electricity in town but it was limited to a few hours in the evening, from 6:00 to 10:00 p.m. The nearest hospital was the government provincial hospital in Tuguegarao, Cagayan. This was 60 kilometers away and could easily be reached by car in one hour. It was fine for referring serious cases that needed specialized treatment although patients, if they were going to be referred, wanted to be taken to Baguio City or Manila.

The early days of my private venture in this part of Kalinga-Apayao, put me right away to a test. I did not have any surgical equipment at that time.

During the first few days in Tabuk, we visited some villages to introduce myself and make it known that there was a physician in town. One Sunday afternoon, just three days after our arrival, a patient was waiting for us when we came home from village visitations.

This was a case of strangulated hernia. He had a lump coming out on and off in his right groin for some time. He had an incarcerated hernia eight hours before coming to our clinic. He did not want to go to the provincial hospital in Tuguegarao for treatment. We told him we had very few instruments, and if we operated on him and found his hernia to be gangrenous, he would have to be referred to the provincial hospital. He insisted that we treat him.

I tried to reduce the hernia but failed. Afterwards, I decided to open up his right groin.

We put him on an ordinary dining table and put around him a small surgical drape used for minor cases. I gave him Demerol and infiltrated the area with local anesthetic. I used two small forceps which were the only instruments available and a new ordinary Gillette blade. These were soaked in antiseptic for a few minutes. I slit the huge bulge. I guess I was lucky; there were no signs of gangrene. The color of the trapped bowels was pinkish,

Forty-eight hours after the operation, he told me and my wife that he was very poor and he did not have money for transportation to Tuguegarao nor could he pay me. We understood that. He was ready to recover at home. We let him go without charging him anything. He came back after seven days to have the stitches removed. There was no sign of infection noted.

The compensation came later. His work was ferrying people across the wide river in a small raft, although his earning was barely enough to buy salt and rice for his family. We learned that he was telling patients to come to me.

A year later, we saw him again but we did not bother to collect a centavo from him. I was happy that he was thankful for what I did to him. To give him peace of mind, we wrote off his debt.

A few years later, his farm yielded a good harvest and he gave us two sacks of rice.

I felt very pleased.

27

THE CLAIRVOYANT

For quite some time I had wanted to have a convincing "reading" by a genuine clairvoyant. I was not impressed by the readings I've had during the last two decades by psychics in Sydney. Their names were advertised in the papers or recommended by friends or patients who had interest in the psychic world but their readings did not impress me. One day, in May 1984, a patient of mine told me about a good clairvoyant. Her name is Pam P.

I went to see her and had a reading. She read my right palm first then compared it with the left, and later, the Tarot cards. She read my past, and every important major event that took place in my life by putting her finger on the lines of my hands. The clairvoyant verified what she had seen by feeling the pulse in my wrist. The "information" made it clearer. According to her, it was for me to believe or not, but the information was relayed to her by her psychic mind, the window by which the paranormal levels could be perceived. She told me during the first part of the "reading" that I have not "thanked Mary." Later, when I was home I realized that my going to Medical School, my guidance of my mission work in northern Luzon was after all the spiritual guidance of an angel named Mary. Was she the mother of Jesus?

The inner urge to search for truth or knowledge of the mystical had been with me since I was 20 years of age. Now, it has been fulfilled. I found the "gifted" person. I was satisfied with her psychic powers of clairvoyance.

I was amazed at the accuracy of her reading. How could she know all the past events in my life? We never met before and I grew up in another country. She had no knowledge of my past.

I was 47 years of age and had many strange encounters before I met Mrs. Pam P. Perhaps, those strange episodes led me to a personal search for the mysterious level of the unknown.

I was fascinated by this window of the metaphysical world. How come the other clairvoyants did not present accurate psychic revelations? It was only Mrs. Pam P who had really impressed me. Perhaps the other clairvoyants did not develop their gifts to the maximum.

Did Mrs. Pam P reveal exact information to others too? Or was it only to me that the psychic world revealed a perfect sequence of happenings so that the lingering doubts I had would be answered? What made me seek the cause and purpose of unnatural phenomena that I experienced? A lot of individuals are charmed by these paranormal events. There are just as many, if not more, of the opposite -- they abhor mystical disclosures.

I asked Mrs. Pam P whose voice communicated with me when I was 20 while in college". She said, 'It was the Holy Ghost.' She added, 'And He is watching you every minute of the day. And there is another angel keeping watch over you.'

In another reading, I asked who the other angel was and the information said "Michael." I searched who this Michael was, and found that he is 'The Lord of The Way.'

In the same reading I asked about the "Holy Ghost" that she had mentioned earlier in my last reading. And she answered, "Elijah!" Can this be true? Or is it the devil answering my question?

The Holy Ghost is one of the posts by which the doctrine of Trinity was conceived. That is – the Father, the Son, and the Holy Ghost. But the concept of the Trinity was only formed centuries after the crucifixion of Jesus Christ. Elijah is the Holy Ghost?! Probably the Ghost of Elijah is holy but he was not part of the Trinity. If this is true, then the Trinity concept is wrong. To me, whether one believes in the Trinity or not, the important thing is that one, rich or poor, gives some concern, a little love, or even more, day by day, towards his fellow man and that he walks humbly with his God.

In one of Mrs. Pam P's readings in 1985, I asked about the appearance of Jesus Christ in the cloud that happened on the eve of my 48th birthday. She blurted out: 'His face was dripping with blood.' Of course it was not real blood! The figure in the cloud that I saw with thorns around his crown was looking down on me as if blood was dripping from his forehead and temples. Mrs. Pam P.s answer verified Jesus' appearance before me.

After a few more readings, I was entirely convinced about the existence of the psychic world. This inspired me to read more about clairvoyance, automatic writing, and the related psychic sciences.

On one occasion, I brought my mother to this clairvoyant. My mother did not believe in psychic matters. When the clairvoyant told her of an event that only she knew, she was amazed. She could not say anything for a few minutes in her bewilderment. The clairvoyant told her that when my father died, just before he was placed in his coffin, Mama put on his feet an old pair of shoes, one of which had a hole in the front sole which he wore for many years. The clairvoyant saw the hole in the shoe.

In year 1985, I became inspired and I started to write about my strange life experiences but gave it up as I was discouraged because my written English was terrible. I had my last reading in August 1987 and the information said, 'Keep it there and it will grow.' I kept what I had written out of sight for many years and before I knew it, I bought a Personal Computer, and began to rewrite my manuscript.

If the past could well be told, then the future could be previewed. (Just as John, the visionary, when he was in exile in the island of Patmos when he wrote the Revelation -- had a preview of the future.) Indeed, I found this accurate. There was "information" given to me that foretold my future events. They came true.

One example is my separation and divorce from my wife. My friends, patients, and I never really thought that I could leave my family. I was told earlier that I would meet someone with a "light complexion" and "by age 52 I shall be married again." Mrs. Pam P added, 'It is a soul reunion and you will be married legally.'

Indeed, after two years I fell deeply in love with another woman and we got married. I had divorced my wife earlier because we could get on well. We were screaming at each other. Where did love go?

Who am I? Who was my previous entity? 'You are a very old soul,' said the information. Past major incarnations were revealed to me. I was over-awed by my past. What cycles of incarnation I had had no bearing or connection with all the different experiences or lifetimes I had and my present existence. This life experience has no recollection or connection with anything I used to be in the past. What had happened in the previous incarnation belongs to the past. This lifetime is an experience of its own.

I have read stories of some hypnotists putting patients into deep hypnotic trances and going back in time, a hundred or 500 years earlier. A lot of hypnotists have had experiences of this nature. They seem to develop some reluctance when they delve further into the subconscious mind of patients. Is it private? I will not be surprised if a book comes out written by hypnotists on the past experiences of some individuals under hypnosis. Somehow they are hesitant because of criticism from their medical colleagues.

I was told that in one of my life experiences I was the apostle Thomas, the doubter. That was engaging! I know that many Christian churches and denominations do not believe in reincarnation. Although I was exposed to the teachings of Christ since I was small, I must admit I am a strong believer in reincarnation. When I attend church services and hear the minister deliver his sermon, something at the back of my mind would not accept what he preaches. Would you believe that "a little bird told me?" This is the reason why during the last 30 years I seldom attended worship services except in baptisms, weddings, and funerals.

There is a mistaken belief that the soul can incarnate into the flesh of animals. This is not true and can never happen. The soul will never enter the womb or flesh of animals.

I have not seen Mrs. Pam P for 30 years now, but all the things she predicted came true during those 30 years. They just happened. Things that I thought would not happen happened unexpectedly.

Years passed and these predictions were forgotten, and then abruptly they came back. What matters is, though seemingly irrelevant the information given were, they happened. They were made known to me many years before their occurrence. I cannot remember the exact date the predictions came true, but the fact is they were "written in the palm of my hands."

We have our destiny, and every human being in his present experience has his own destiny written in the fine prints of his hands, some of them distinguished only by supernatural beings. My Karma is likewise written in the lines of my palm. 'The prints in your hands are just so clear,' as Mrs. Pam P said.

People should not condemn, nor be scared of, nor discard, psychic phenomena. If the future is foretold they should not be afraid, but they should be prepared to meet the prediction head on. At times, people's religious background prevents them from getting involved. However, time changes. Should we not adapt to these time changes?

Today, there are many clairvoyants or psychic astrologers. A psychic medium can create a connection between you and the unseen world of energy that exists around you. Many dedicated psychic mediums devote their lives to helping others who are lost and unhappy. But many make money out of their gifts.

28

THE SPIRIT THAT WOKE ME!

The brother of my wife who was 13 at the time, went with me to Manila to purchase surgical equipment and other supplies. Driving from Tabuk to Manila and back in my old Chrysler (1951 model) and deprived me of 24 hours of sleep. At that time the provincial roads were in a shocking state. From Tabuk to Baguio City were large "moon holes" or craters almost every few meters. It took us ten hours to navigate these two places. The old highway from Baguio City to Manila was much better but it took us another six hours of driving.

We did our shopping the whole day, and drove back to Baguio in the evening. It was midnight when I almost had a head-on collision with a bus on the MacArthur highway.

I was tired but continued to drive. I must have dozed off for a few seconds and woke up suddenly and found my car occupying the wrong lane of the highway.

I immediately swerved back to my lane and the oncoming bus missed me by an inch or two. All I heard was the bus honking as it whizzed past me, and the air waves made my car vibrate strongly as if it had been splashed by an ocean wave. The bus must have been traveling at 120 kph or more. This was not unusual at this time of the night. That shook me and I was fully awake again.

Ten or 20 minutes later, I felt drowsy again. I thought of pulling over as soon as I found a nice spot. Before I knew it, I dozed off again, only to be awakened when my head flicked forward, and I found myself occupying the other side of the highway. I swerved to the right instantly. Just then another bus traveling at high speed missed my car. Another one or two seconds and we could have been smashed to death. All the while Jerry was sleeping like a log.

It must have been the same spirit that saved me twice. Today, a lot of vehicular accidents happen because the driver would doze off and hit or be hit by another car or dive into a deep ravine.

I pulled over and slept at the side of the road. Two hours of sleep should be enough.

When I woke up I realized I had slept for six hours. Jerry had been awake for some time and was throwing pebbles 20 meters away under the stream of bright morning light. He never knew what happened some hours back.

29

GLUED TO MY WORK

A few months passed in Tabuk and Luke, my second son, was born on the same improvised table that I used to do the hernia repair.

We already had a name for our clinic – St. Luke's Clinic. my wife, had finished her nursing course at St. Luke's Hospital in Quezon City, and she liked the idea of naming our second son after her alma mater too.

We were still far from acquiring much needed instruments. We needed an operating table, an autoclave, a suction machine, lamps, surgical drapes and gowns. A generator for lighting principally the operating room was considered primary and other supplies needed for major surgical cases followed. So far, major surgical cases were referred elsewhere except emergency Cesarean Operations and forceps for deliveries. I no longer thought of going abroad.

Two months after my second son was born, the brother of my wife and I went to Manila. This was the time I almost died twice, were it not for the supernatural spirit who saved me. When Jerry and I were in Manila, we bought surgical instruments and a delivery table (which we also used for major operations).

We acquired a second-hand generator a few weeks later. For some time (before we acquired the needed instruments), I was contented doing obstetrical deliveries, forceps, and Caesarean Sections with a kerosene lantern, a flashlight for back-up (when we had emergency C/S at night), suction, and two 200 ml irrigation syringes.

The first operating room we had was an old bedroom. It measured three and a half meters wide and five meters long. It was on the first floor of a two story-house we rented.

In this room, we did an innumerable number of obstetrical cases the next 12 months. After a year, we bought the house and the adjacent lot. I drew the plans for a 25-bed emergency hospital, which we later named St. Luke's Emergency Hospital.

Of the four children we had, I delivered three. My first child by Caesarean Section on the 28th of August 1968. My second son was delivered normally on the 14th of September 1969. My third child (a daughterP on the 18th of October 1971 was delivered in Abatan Lutheran Hospital. This was seven years after I treated some patients and delivered babies in the same Lutheran Clinic while on summer vacation from medical school and collecting insects in the wild of Abatan for Bishop Museum of Hawaii.

My wife had a difficult time with the delivery of my third child. Her uterus did not contract after delivery (uterine inertia), and she developed post-partum hemorrhage. She received a total of 10 ampoules of Pitocin before her uterus responded. Hysterectomy would have to be performed. At the last minute, the uterus contracted. The second name of my daughteer is **Cin**ia, as a reminder of the ten ampoules of Pito**cin** the mother was given.

I had planned to attend Nellie's delivery that day but my replacement, the replacement physician did not arrive in Tabuk on time. I could not leave behind serious patients. The following day I could not drive to Abatan either as I was not able to sleep for 24 hours because of delivering three babies the previous night. The following day I could not take a rest as I had to attend to the daily average of 30 patients and admissions.

My fourth child (another daughter) was delivered by elective Caesarean Section on the 19th of March 1974 after two interruptions. An emergency Caesarean Section interrupted my wife's elective procedure. Later in the afternoon as she was being prepared, another case for emergency Caesarean was brought in. Finally she had her turn that evening.

Since we moved to Tabuk, I was glued to my work. In five years I gained a wealth of clinical and surgical experiences on my own initiative. The plan to go abroad was long abandoned. Of course, the bits of surgical skill I developed were really nothing compared with the skills my school contemporaries learned from specialized training abroad. Nonetheless I was happy in my work -- at our own hospital in Tabuk.

In 1975, I had the chance to take a short course in Anesthetics at the Philippine General Hospital in Manila. The Medicare system in the Philippines at that time required a physician who administered anesthesia and performed operations as a surgeon at the same time to secure a Certificate in Anesthesia so he can claim the Social Security System and GSIS payments of patients who were members of the social security systems. Teachers and officials and employees of government and private establishments were covered by Medicare.

After six months, I finished the course in PGH. I was able to give GA (General Anesthesia) to some surgical cases. I did the intubations, using Halothane, and when the patient was stabilized a nurse did the bagging (pumping of air and oxygen via a bag) and monitoring of vital signs and intravenous fluids while the operation or exploration was going on.

There were a lot gunshot wounds, stabbings and motor vehicle accidents in the area. Patients preferred local or epidural anesthesia as they were afraid of GA. When a case could not be done with epidural, GA had to be used. Most patients were scared of Ether. This was because during and after World War II Ether anesthesia was used in most hospitals and a big number of deaths were attributed to Ether. Ensuing vomiting and aspiration led to severe pneumonia and death in nearby government hospitals. But with the advent of newer GA, mortality no longer became a threat.

I learned a lot of practical skills in my practice in the rural areas. After some exposure, a rural doctor can easily diagnose a case by asking the patient a few questions, looking at his face or body, and pressing his fingertips. In recent years, residents and doctors in big hospitals make their diagnoses based on laboratory examinations (blood), X-rays, ultrasounds and scans, and the latest MRI. Medicine has advanced tremendously — in the cities, at least.

At our clinic, we had meager laboratory facilities, but our trained pharmacist and a laboratory technician did a magnificent job of making-do with available instruments.

Malignant cases or other difficult maladies were referred to Baguio City or Manila.

The risk that doctors took when they practiced in rural areas was high: they could die from gunshot wounds as the police and lawless elements exchange fire. One evening, during a town fiesta or festival, three policemen spotted a wanted man. Bullets flew all over the place. One policeman died instantly. He was our neighbor. The wanted man, who had a gunshot wound, rushed to my office at about seven o'clock in the evening, his left hand pressing the upper left side of his abdomen. He poked a revolver between my eyes. He said, 'I just shot a police officer, will you treat me?'

'Of course,' I answered, 'Only if you put the gun down!' He obliged. Would he have shot me if I refused? What could I do? Somehow I had the feeling he would not shoot me.

While I was operating on this wanted man, somebody tried to finish him off from outside the window of the clinic. He aimed his M-15 rifle at the patient, but could not fire as I was moving right or left of the patient. The trigger man, who was a relative of the dead cop, could not pull the trigger. "Don't do it! You might hit the doctor!" His companion said. I was told of this the next day. The wanted man was transferred to the Philippine Constabulary compound two days later and I followed up his case in the barracks.

By 1975, there were a few clinics in the area. The government hospital had opened in Bulanao, six kilometers from my clinic.

For six years I was glued to my work. I worked day in and day out seven days a week until I was able to have another doctor working with me. Nellie was tireless. She took charge of the nursing side and cleaning section. She was assisting me in the operating room most of the time.

30

DONE TO THE LEAST
OF MY BRETHREN!

An unforgettable surgical incident happened on a Sunday, sometime in 1972.
My wife, three children and I were getting ready for church. We saw a number of people carrying a patient in an improvised hammock made of a large thick blanket suspended on a bamboo pole. They were in a hurry. Some distance away a flock followed.

"Oh, oh, trouble. I can smell it. It looks like the Lord does not want me to go to church!" I talked loudly to myself. For some time I had not gone to church.

Even before the woman was transferred to the emergency trolley, I had the feeling this patient had placenta previa. The hammock was dripping fresh blood. She was extremely pale from blood loss. And she was still bleeding profusely!

"This is the third bleeding episode," the husband claimed. "She is on her eighth month of gestation. She bled two weeks ago and a week ago but they were not heavy. This time the bleeding would not stop.

I did not ask him anything. He gave the information quite fast.

He and his companions did not know what placenta previa was. An angry thought was in my mind.

"You should have brought her the first time she bled."

I was emphatic. It was too late. If I had advised her complete rest in the hospital and an elective Caesarean operation was carried out, the chance of my advice being followed was almost nil.

The patient was ghostly pale. Almost all her blood was drained out. She was extremely weak, gasping for breath, unable to say a word or move her limb. Her eyes would not open. Her carotid pulse was very faint. Her BP could not be read. She was almost dead!

I examined her abdomen and felt the movement of the baby in the womb. She was immediately wheeled into the delivery room, and without saying anything to the husband, I put on a pair of surgical gloves, grabbed the scalpel, and cut her abdomen. There was no anesthesia infiltrated. The patient did not feel anything. She was numb all over. A sudden thought came to my mind: "This happened before when I was an intern in Labor Hospital." The memory came flooding back to me. I could remember well what happened before. Now -- I was the one holding the scalpel.

The operation was practically bloodless except for an insignificant trace of dark venous blood when I cut through the womb. I pulled the baby out of the womb quickly. The baby was extremely purple. He gave a weak movement. I handed the baby to the nurse beside me and then extracted the placenta. I closed the uterus and the abdomen quickly. Through the patient's thin-skinned groin an 18-Gauge needle was inserted to the femoral vein. As soon as I got the femoral vein, I ordered, 'Pump the plasma expander!' Meanwhile the nurse was busy resuscitating the baby. As soon as he gave a faint cry the blue baby started to change color slowly. This became better with oxygen flowing into his lungs.

The mother was unconscious. As the plasma expander flowed fast into her veins the vital signs started to pick up. I could feel her pulse. I followed this up with intravenous fluids at full blast and with the aid of an oxygen mask.

'She might live,' I exclaimed to the people in the room.

I rushed out of the delivery room and with a clear voice demanded: 'Who will donate blood?' There were possibly 20 people in the room.

Everybody was silent. Not a tongue moved.

'Oh, no, not this group!' I moaned.

'No, she cannot have blood,' the husband responded. 'You see, we belong to the Jehovah's Witness religion.'

For a second I thought I should not argue with them.

'If one or two can give blood, I am sure she will live.' I was insistent. Of course she needed more than 4 liters of blood.

'No! No! It is against our religion!'

'Is it your religion or your God?' I countered. 'Go to your pastor now and I will talk to him.'

Nobody moved. They stood at the corners of the room, waiting for the patient to claim her fate that was not for her to take but for them to prolong a life but were banned by their religious belief. I had contributed my share to save her life and she was hanging by a thread to get the share from her family or friends.

'Her fate is in your hands!' my voice was like a preacher's.

'Do what you can do but no blood. That oxygen is enough. If God takes her life, it is His Will.' The husband was the only one who was able to say something.

This was a cold-hearted response! And everybody present was dumb. No one could say anything.

'Is it not that God gave us talent that we should use properly?' I sounded like an evangelist.

There was no answer. A long minute passed. The waiting was too long. I was talking to a brick wall. It would have been easier to get a response from a leaf as it swayed its answer when the wind blew.

The patient's pulse became very faint again. Her BP was inaudible.

'Remember Jesus when He said, 'If you have done this to the least of my brethren, you have done this unto me?' I tried once more, hoping against hope that they will understand what I said. They understood what I meant, but they did not listen.

The husband and everybody in the flock remained still. If this woman died . . . My thoughts faded as she clutched a few moments of her life unable to understand what was going on. Or maybe she understood. She had a tear in each eye.

Twenty minutes passed since I started trying to convince anyone to donate that precious blood. The patient stared blankly at the ceiling. Her eyes became fixed. Then the heartbeat was gone. Tears trickled down her cheeks. Did she understand what I meant?

This was the church service I meant to attend that morning!

It was beyond my understanding how Jehovah's Witnesses even today deny life when something could be done to prolong life. The significance of the blood is that of atoning death. Meaning that by following the pattern Jesus set we reconcile with God. This is the belief in some Christian denominations.

Blood transfusions have saved countless lives. Is it God's Will that this religious sect should not receive blood? Is it really against His Will? Or is it the indoctrination of whoever started this church?

One of the greatest advances in the medical field today is the transplant of human organs. Are these not man's endowment to mankind? All along it is man's will to discover God-given wisdom and understanding.

Letting a person die when something can be done is a rebellion against the Creator. Nobody is to blame if every effort and talent had been rendered and nothing comes out of it. This is the reason why a lot of researches are being made to heal diseases and prolong life.

Biblically speaking, the Good Samaritan is an example of prolonging life.

The episode that happened that particular Sunday morning always reminded me of Jesus speaking to Peter just before He ascended: 'If you have done this to the least of my brethren, you have done it unto Me.'

I did my part. A greater part, I suppose. All that was needed was "Yes" and I could have rounded up a few persons who would be willing to donate blood. If my blood matched with hers, I would have given her my blood.

That purple baby was a four-year-old little girl when I left Tabuk. She did not have brain damage after all.

What have they done to the mother of this little girl?

31

THE FAST RIDE HOME TO TABUK

I had an assistant in the later part of 1973. My usual 24 hours call daily became every other day. Some weekends I was free and I could spend a little time with the kids.

One day I went down to Manila via Baguio City with the two boys, Ike and Luke in our Volkswagen van. The children had a great time. They saw Manila for the first time and they were amazed at the tall buildings and places of interest, especially the animals at the Manila zoo.

The weather was gloomy when we left Manila. The waves on Roxas Boulevard in Manila Bay smashed heavily against the concrete walls, and the tall coconuts tress were swaying from the gusty winds. We planned to go home leisurely through Baguio City and sleep overnight at at the sister of my wife.

I had forgotten to monitor the weather earlier otherwise had we known a typhoon was on its way we could have started much earlier and heed for home. The plan changed when we heard on the car radio that a typhoon was hitting northern Luzon in 12 hours. This was a strong typhoon with predicted winds of 180 kph.

I pressed on the accelerator as soon as I heard the broadcast. We drove non-stop. I knew the terrain in the mountain provinces. If we got delayed we would be trapped for days by landslides along the mountain highway. We did not make a stopover in Baguio but proceeded to Tabuk.

Sixty kilometers away from Tabuk, at Lubuagan, the typhoon raged. Trees started to fall on the road and occasionally rocks rolled down the mountain sides and blocked the roads. We were roughly about 20 kilometers away from Tabuk when I saw from the rear window of my van a huge landslide cutting off the road. We just made it in a few seconds. ***Is it not*** *strange that after traveling for many hours it took only a few seconds for us to pass that point of the road and then a huge landslide came down?*

It may be a coincidence, but somehow the three of us were lucky. Tabuk was isolated for one month. Transportation by bus was at a standstill. Many were trapped and had to hike long distances to get to where they were going.

It was not the strong winds that bothered me most. The path of the biggest and longest river in the Philippines was to be feared because the flood could change the course of the river, and the small hospital that I built without any subsidy might be carried away.

It was spared!

32

THE HANDS THAT LOCKED!

In 1974 I had a most frightful near- death-claiming incident.

The members of my family had gone to Sagada two days earlier for a family reunion. Sagada was 120 kilometers north of Tabuk by-passing Lubuagan town and Bontoc. The road between Lubuagan and Bontoc was the most terrifying and dangerous road in northern Luzon that I had traversed. The road was built before World War II and became deteriorated with time. The traffic was one way in some segments and there were waiting "gates" in between to allow one car to go through while other vehicles waited for their turn. It can take a few hours for one to reach one's destination. To make a wider road along the 70 kilometers of granite mountain wall would be very costly for the government.

I went to Sagada the next day with two friends as the other physician did not come up on time to relieve me. There were two deliveries and one C/S that night. There were nights we were not busy, but at other times patients came one after the other. It had to happen that night!

Robbed of sleep, we started at six o'clock in the morning in my Old Plymouth sedan. My travelling companions were, my trustworthy mason, and the sister of my pharmacist, a schoolteacher.

We formed a convoy of two buses, a jeepney and two cars. Travelling in convoys was the safe thing to do as there were hold-uppers armed with modern weapons on the mountain highway. Half of the time, the convoy waited for 20 or 30 minutes in between gates. There were 13 gates and the distance between gates ranged from seven to 20 kilometers.

My hands became numb after three hours of driving slowly in this dangerous road. I slowed down at a curve where there was enough room for the convoy to pass through. I let them go ahead because I wanted to rest my numb hands. I never experienced this numbness before. Was it due to lack of sleep?

Driving the last few kilometers towards Bontoc seemed difficult. I was making a turn at a curve when both my forearms and hands locked suddenly. I could not move or lift or release both my hands from the steering wheel. The car was going to dive into the cliff!

It happened suddenly as I made an acute turn over a bend overlying a deep canyon. I could not undo my grips. My left forearm was crossed over the right. Both forearms and hands were frozen! Lifeless! The steering wheel became fixed. I could not think of anything. My mind became blank. We were going straight into the deep precipice. This was more than a thousand feet.

At the last second, my right foot just stepped on the brake. This was probably a reflex reaction. My friends were asleep. I woke them up, telling them to move very slowly because we were hanging by the edge of the cliff.

Peding slowly got out of the car and checked the front tires. One tire was hanging by the edge but the other was still on solid ground. Two more inches and we would have gone spinning down. My mason placed large rocks in front of the tires to prevent the car's moving forward. I did not get out of the car. I was afraid that if I released the brakes the car might keel over.

Then, I reversed very slowly.

Six hours later, we were drinking beer in Sagada, but my mason's knees were still shaking!

'Were you not afraid of the incident? This incident almost sent us to our graves?' He asked.

'A little,' I answered.

However, I thanked my "spirit guides" silently for saving our lives.

33

THE TWIST IN MY DESTINY

In May 1976, I was a delegate to the International Family Planning Program sponsored by the Inter-Church Commission on Medical Care (ICCMC). The convention was supposed to be in Houston, Texas, U.S.A. My plane ticket had been purchased by ICCMC but the US Embassy in Manila refused to give me a visa per memorandum of President Ferdinand Marcos. My name had appeared in the embassy's list of passers of the ECFMG (Educational Council for Foreign Medical Graduates). President Marcos banned doctors who had passed the exam from leaving for the U.S. This was done reportedly because Filipino physicians and recent medical graduates who passed the ECFMG could easily find residency training in the U.S. and do not return to the Philippines.

To make use of the plane ticket and enjoy a one month vacation, I had to fly out of the Philippines. China, Hongkong and Singapore were suggested. My sister, who used to work with the **Manila Bulletin**, now with **The Philippine Star** where she is a columnist, suggested Australia. I liked that. I went to the Australian Embassy which gave me a visa in no time.

I had no intention of staying long in Australia as I had my small hospital in Tabuk to take care of. My family and patients would be waiting for me. However, a good physician and surgeon, took my place for 12 months whenever or wherever I went away. He could do the medical and surgical tasks if I stayed in Australia for some time.

On the 26th of May 1976 my plane landed at the Mascot International Airport in Sydney.

"Did you come in to die?" The taxi driver asked me.

"I beg your pardon?"

He knew I just came out of the international airport. Why should he ask me that question?

He pronounced today as "to die."

Goodness me, why should anybody think that I came to Australia to die? I found out later that the pronunciation of some words in Australia was very different from the American pronunciation. I never thought the sound of English would be very different in this part of the world. That showed ignorance when one has not travelled out of the country.

The taxi driver brought me to Travelodge, Darlinghurst. I walked for a few hours that afternoon to acquaint myself with the new environment. The city was certainly very clean and beautiful unlike the dirty and polluted cities in the Philippines.

The following morning (Sunday), I got up early to see interesting places. I noticed that at 7 in the morning, the streets were empty. Where was everybody? At that hour in Manila, even on Sundays, the streets were already busy and noisy — with passenger jeepneys and buses honking every minute.

I looked at a sign in one corner that said, "NO STANDING." That intrigued me. Maybe one could crawl. Why would they not allow people to stand? I kept on walking because standing was not allowed. A few persons walked down the street at nine in the morning. (That was in 1976 but now at this time, there would be a crowd). I saw another sign "NO STANDING" sign, but somebody was leaning on the signpost. Later I realized that sign was for buses, meaning—NO PARKING.

The third day, I got bored. Reading the newspapers and watching black and white television in the hotel did not alleviate my boredom. There were several ads in the newspapers that attracted my attention. They invited applicants for Resident Medical Officers; at the time I learned there was a big demand for RMOs throughout New South Wales. The temptation to answer the ads got hold of me. The next day I decided to apply for a position in a few hospitals. Who knows I might be accepted. I came to Australia mainly to see places. On the other hand a lot of new things could be learned.

I went to Wollongong about 120 kilometers south of Sydney. I had an interview for a position as a resident medical officer. After the interview, a requirement was needed. They needed my Medical Registration Number. I was told to go first to the Medical Board at Macquarie Street in Sydney. There were many requirements and I did not have my Diploma or papers from the Medical School I graduated. The only evidence that I was a medical graduate was a photocopy of my ECFMG (Educational Council for Foreign Medical Graduates) sponsored by USA which stated I had passed this examination.

Walking down the main street of Wollongong, I met a well-dressed Asian.

"Are you a Filipino?" He inquired in Tagalog.

"Do I look like Japanese?" I answered with a smile.

After a few minutes of jolly conversation, he invited me to go back to Sydney with him. He introduced me to a few Filipino families. The family of M. and F. S was very accommodating. The head of the family asked me to move to his rented apartment in Redfern.

They got my travelling bag at the hotel and settled me comfortably in their home. They told their life stories. Many of the Filipino families came from war-torn Vietnam, some from the Middle East. I told them briefly my background.

On the fifth day, I was restless. I told Mars that if I applied for work in a hospital for a few weeks, and was accepted, that would be great. He encouraged me. I borrowed his typewriter and sent applications to a few hospitals. The next day, I received a telegram from Coffs Harbour asking me to report for an interview. He was the Medical Superintendent of Coffs Harbour District Hospital. Coffs Harbour was about 600 kilometers north of Sydney. I took the "Red Train" that night from Central Station. The interview was brief. Dr. Winton asked me if I could start the next day. I told him I had to go back to Sydney to register at the Medical Board of New South Wales.

At the Medical Board on Macquarie Street, I informed them that I had an interview with the Medical Superintendent in Coffs Harbour District Hospital and I was accepted. The Medical Superintendent wanted me to start right away. The Officer-in-Charge (at the Immigration Department) phoned the Medical Superintendent for verification. He took down my name and asked me to send my curricula and other data. I was allowed to work with a temporary license.

A telegram was sent to my wife to send my diploma and all my medical school records. My wife and the children were happy. I had assured them I would be back in six months. My temporary replacement, in Tabuk was doing fine.

I started work at Coff's Harbour District Hospital. When I received all the needed papers, I went back to the Medical Board. The twist of my destiny had happened. I had not planned for this. Somebody "up there" must be kind to me.

Working in a 100-bed District Hospital in Australia during the first year with consultants around and with complete laboratory facilities was very pleasant and educational. The population of Coffs Harbour at that time was 27,000. I acquired more knowledge in medicine. This new exposure was completely different from the experiences I had amongst the poor people in the Philippines. It seemed nobody was poor in Australia, comparatively speaking.

There were five RMOs rotating in Casualty (A & E), assisting surgeons when they did their rounds in the wards, and the ICU. I thoroughly enjoyed my work but after six months, my conscience bothered me. Finally, I told the Medical Superintendent that I was an overstaying visitor.

'Are you willing to stay in Australia?' he asked.

'Of course, I do. Life here is a lot better compared to where I worked in the Philippines.' I did not tell him, though, that I experienced some degree of discrimination in the hospital. In time, many of the hospital personnel became my friends except for a couple of RMOs who seemed jealous of me because patients who knew me asked for me and not them. These two were Caucasian co-residents who did not want to do anything with me but find fault.

"You are my Super-resident, and you work hard," Dr. Winton told me.

I felt embarrassed about this, thinking that some people were calling me "Jungle Doctor." But I did not mind that because it was true. Maybe they have not heard of Dr. Tom Dooley or Albert Schweitzer.

The Medical Superintendent asked for my passport and phoned the Immigration Department. I heard him talk to Immigration Officer, saying that Coffs Harbour District Hospital needed me badly as a Resident Medical Officer. The Immiragtion Officer told him to send my passport to Immigration Office at Chifley Square.

In two weeks, my passport came back by mail, stamped "Permanent Resident." Somebody 'up there' must like me! I was very thankful to Dr. Winton and the channels involved in processing my status so I could stay permanently in Australia.

In February 1977, my wife and the two girls, joined me in Coffs Harbour. The two boys joined us a year later. I had a new job in Parramatta.. I was worked at Parramatta District Hospital for 18 months.

There were 200 foreign medical graduates who took the medical and oral examinations. We were informed later that only 5 per cent passed.

I was lucky to be one of the 5 per cent.

34

START OF MY GENERAL PRACTICE IN SYDNEY

After passing the New South Wales oral and written examination (AMEC) for foreign medical graduates, I worked for 18 months at the Parramatta District Hospital, a 400-bed general hospital, as a Senior Medical Officer, rotating in all major fields of Medicine and Surgery. I rotated every three months, from Intensive Care, to Anesthetics, to Orthopedics, Medical Department, Obstetrics and Gynecology to Casualty (A & E) and the Out-Patient Department. I was interested in all of these assignments, but best of all in the Accident and Emergency section as this reminded me of the kinds of trauma I had encountered in my early years of practice in the hinterlands of northern Luzon. I did not do any operations in Parramatta, but I was the one who called the surgeons on duty and sometimes assisted some of them.

One night, an elderly patient was brought to the hospital by ambulance. He had an acute obstruction of his penis. On examination he had severe phimosis and the tip of the foreskin was totally closed up. He said he had been dribbling for weeks when he passed water. I asked him if his penis would balloon every time he tried to empty his urine. He answered, 'Yes.'

I did circumcision right away under local anesthesia. He went home after two hours. There was no complication.

The following morning, the Surgical Superintendent, came to me. "I heard you did circumcision under LA last night." I answered that circumcision was a routine task for me in the Philippines, usually during Easter time. Some would ask a barber or somebody who was known to do circumcision to do it under a guava tree, with only a kitchen knife for instrument and pressed guava leaves to speed up healing of the incision.

"When you have a case like that next time can you call me?" He asked me. "I have not done one under local anesthesia."

We used to do a lot of circumcision with babies without anesthesia at the Nursery in Parramatta District Hospital. The babies were only a few days old. This is banned now. As to the reason why? I do not know. Circumcision is not only a Jewish practice; it is done in other countries like the Philippines as a cultural practice.

My name was written on the Register of Medical Practitioners in New South Wales on the fourth day of April 29, 1979.

In October 1979, I resigned from Parramatta District Hospital to set up my own practice in Blacktown, New South Wales, a suburb in the western area of Sydney. The Medical Superintent would not release me at first. He discouraged me from practicing in Blacktown, because, he said, there were many good General Practitioners in the area I would be penniless in six months. This did not discourage me. However, I was very grateful to him and the assistant Medical Superintendent, for the job and training the district hospital gave me.

From the jungles of northern Luzon, I was now a General Practitioner in a foreign land.

35

HOPE GIVEN UP!

While in private practice for a couple of months in Blacktown, a nurse I knew from the Intensive Care Unit of Parramatta District Hospital called me. Sister M. was the night matron and she told me that Cecilia L. (once a night matron) was in ICU. I worked with Cecilia in the Casualty Section of Parramatta District Hospital for 6 months and we became close friends.

I was told she collapsed in the hospital toilet and when she was found she was markedly cyanotic (very blue). She developed respiratory arrest followed by cardiac arrest. She was known to have a lot of allergies. It could have been an acute bronchospasm that triggered it. The doctors were able to resuscitate her. Then she was placed on the artificial ventilator known as IPPR (Intermittent Respiratory Positive Pressure) for many days.

She was in coma for seven days. EEG was done. This showed a flat record, meaning she would be a vegetable if she recovered. The nurses, doctors, and the director of the Intensive Care Unit believed she would not survive. Everybody gave up on her! On the sixth day, I visited her. I felt sad seeing a good friend unconscious, ventilated by the IPPR apparatus.

I touched Mrs. C. L. feet and words just came out of my mouth: "You will live and walk again."

The few nurses around and sister Maroni, the night matron, heard what I said.

'What? What did you say?'

Sister Maroni could not believe what I said. 'You must be crazy!'

The following day, Mrs. C. L. began to move parts of her body. Her breathing became spontaneous and the endotracheal tube was removed.

She gradually gained strength. She walked again and could talk although she could not be understood. The words were all muffled. Her coordination and mental state were very poor. She could not recognize anybody, not even her husband. After a few weeks she was transferred to a private hospital for rehabilitation. I visited her. I was surprised she recognized me right away. I was the first person she recognized. (I remembered my mother when she was recovering from severe malaria during World War II; I was the only one she recognized when she came back from her Near-Death Experience.)

'In due time, you will be normal again,' I assured her.

In a few months she was back to almost normal. She was back at home in a couple of months. She and her husband who was working with General Electric, have been to New York for three years, to Hongkong for one year, and are now back in Australia.

She is enjoying life again. She invited my family in December 2007 to their retirement home in Macquarie, New South Wales.

She still telephones me once a year and tells me she is very well. I talked to her last year, 2012. She remembered everything.

I was very glad she recovered 43 years ago and is alive and well today.

Was the EEG wrong?

Or was this a miracle? This was done by the mystical world! Not me.

36

SLEEP DRIVING?

The first few years of my practice kept me quite busy. I answered home visits in the middle of the night seven days a week. I lost a lot of sleep.

One night, my wife woke me up at 1:00 o'clock in the morning. She said somebody wanted a house call. I changed into my casual clothes, got into my car and drove along the Great Western Highway leading towards Penrith, a western suburb. A lot of cars overtook me. The cars were speeding more than 80 km per hour. I glanced at my speedometer. I was doing only 60 kph.

I stepped on the accelerator. It would not go any faster. I pressed harder; still it would not go any faster. I thought something was wrong. I had been driving for 10 to 15 minutes. Then I asked myself, where am I going? I realized then that I was driving towards another direction. I had to turn back east to Wenworthville where I was supposed to answer the house call. I could speed up then to 80 km per hour.

Did I drive while asleep? If there is sleepwalking then this episode would be sleep driving. Are there reported cases? I wondered why the car would not go more than 60 km an hour. Either my subconscious mind was controlling the driving, or an alien took hold of my motor center. I had total recall of the whole episode whereas in cases of sleepwalking there is no recollection of the event. If I have total recall then it would not be considered sleep driving. What was it? Was I possessed again?

The following week, it happened again. I had to give up night calls before I meet an accident.

37

THE SPIRIT THAT WOKE ME UP AGAIN!

Sometime in July 1983, I went fishing one weekend with friends and my two boys, Ike and Luke. We had fine time fishing at a place known as The Entrance, a small gulf at Gosford, 120 kilometers north of Sydney. We caught a few large silver breams, cooked some catch on the spot in burning charcoal and brought home the rest of the catch the next day. The night out fishing was very relaxing. We did this a number of times.

The following day on this particular weekend, we drove back to Greystanes, the suburb where we had our residence.

Everybody went ahead of us and I took my time driving with my two sons. It was Sunday, mid-morning. The car heater kept us warm and soon after I felt sleepy.

I must have dozed off for two seconds. Suddenly, I was awakened and found myself at the edge of a precipice. There was ample time to step on the brakes. It made my heart jump. My God! We could have fallen down 20 meters into the rocks. I thought of Ike and Luke and I felt bad. Something dreadful could have happened. I started to drive fast to keep myself awake.

Twenty minutes passed and I started to feel drowsy again. I took big breaths and turned up the radio for fast music and dabbed a wet towel on my face so I would not fall asleep. I kept on driving. Before I knew it, I was awakened again, and found myself on the other lane. Luckily, there was no oncoming vehicle. All the while, Ike and Luke were sound asleep.

I could not take any more chances. So, I stopped the car and slept for an hour along the Pacific Highway.

The claws of death almost got the three of us!

38

AN ASTRAL PROJECTION!

Kathy M., an ICU nursing sister at Mr. Druitt Hospital was known to suffer from severe atopic dermatitis and bronchial asthma.

On the 30th of July 1985, she came to my surgery with severe wheezing. She was very pale and off –color.

She had been discharged from the Intensive Care Unit of Mt. Druitt General Hospital a week previous. Kathy worked in that section of the hospital.

According to her she had Aminophyline infusion while admitted in the ICU. At that time Aminophyline was commonly administered for acute bronchospasm. I had used this in the Philippines many times before, mixing it with 50% dextrose.

I gave this intravenous injection to Mrs. K. M. very slowly. As I was giving this her eyes became fixed on the ceiling blankly, and she was not breathing. I tried to get her attention by asking, 'Are you all right?' She did not respond. She was slightly bluish! I felt for her pulse. It was very faint! She was having a respiratory arrest! Should I do mouth- to mouth- resuscitation?

I pressed the emergency alarm and my wife came rushing to the room. I looked for an ampoule of Calcium gluconate and gave it intravenously to her bulging cubital veins. There was no response. Mrs. K. M. was turning more cyanotic (bluish). She would have a cardiac arrest in another minute! I was about to give her a strong blow to her chest when she took a big breath. In two or three minutes she was able to move easily as if nothing had happened.

Five minutes passed. She talked coherently.

I told her what happened.

'I know what happened, I saw everything,' she said.

'I think you have just experienced an astral projection.' I tried to explain what I meant.

'I saw a lady in blue standing at the foot of the examination table,' she said.

She could have seen my wife, Nellie, who was assisting me, but she was dressed in white.

Was this 'Lady in Blue' an angel?

I called the husband and explained to him everything that happened.

She was not in respiratory distress anymore and no appreciable wheezing was heard in her chest.

The husband took her home after 30 minutes with my instruction to call me anytime or bring her to the hospital if I could not be contacted.

When she came for follow-up a week later, the husband said, "She did not cough throughout the week!"

A few years passed and she never had an attack of Bronchial Asthma, and her atopic dermatitis had not flared up.

I believe she had witnessed what we call a near-death phenomenon. This has been reported in many cases of cardiac arrest and patients coming back to life. To me, I still believe that that lady in blue was an angel.

Now I can call the lady in blue an angel who has been assigned to watch over me.

A lot of people don't believe in this phenomenon.

Do you?

39

THE STRANGE RECOGNITION!

Mrs. Doris O., a pleasant elderly at 75, underwent an operation for glaucoma of the right eye in June 1983 at Westmead Centre. The specialist had performed right trabelectomy and reformation of the anterior chamber and drainage of suprachoroidal fluid on her. After the operation, she developed what the doctors termed "organic brain syndrome." She was confined for many days at Westmead Hospital. She did not recognize anybody, not even her son John, who was very close to her, nor her daughter-in-law Beverly. She was totally disoriented as to time and place, and did not even know her name.

Her son and the son's wife were worried that Doris might not recover from this "organic brain syndrome." The doctors who took care of her assumed that her condition might have been caused by the anesthetic gas used during her eye operation.

The daughter-in-law asked me late one afternoon if I could visit her mother-in-law at Westmead Hospital. I did during my lunch break the following day.

The moment I walked into the room, she recognized me! Was there a curtain that was unveiled? Or was it my aura? She had been in the hospital for seven days. The instant I appeared at the door, she explained, 'My doctor!' From that time on she recognized her relatives in the room.

Was this coincidence? As far as I know coincidences don't happen!

Doris passed away in October 1986.

40

IS IT REALLY COINCIDENCE?

To psychics, coincidence or chance or serendipity does not happen. Things happen not by chance but because somewhere out there is a Supernatural Force controlling the complexities of life's existence.

In October 1985, my mother had grown giant-sized dahlias in front of my clinic. They were glorious and very beautiful, some of them colored pink and crimson.

When I opened my clinic at eight o'clock one Monday morning most of the beautiful flowers were pulled out except for the smaller ones still sprouting their young leaves.

How could anybody destroy such beautiful flowers? I felt my adrenaline rushing to my brain. I was angry. I made a "curse" that whoever destroyed the flowers would meet a terrible repercussion "from above." I knew they were pulled out by drug addicts and the tubers sold to the flower nursery to earn a few dollars for their habit.

Three weeks later when the remaining dahlias were in bloom, I placed a distinct sign on the ground close to the flowers: 'WHOEVER WILL DESTROY THESE FLOWERS, WILL MEET HIS OWN DISASTER.'

The next morning all the flowers were pulled out and the tubers too. I knew that whoever did it had seen the sign and ignored it. What a waste of beauty! The magnificent flowers were appreciated by everybody who saw them. Beauty was gone in a stroke.

Two days later I was called to see a woman who lived a block away from my clinic. She was hysterical because her son (who was a drug addict) had been shot in a shoot-out with policemen. The teenager was caught with a stolen car.

Since that time, our flowers were not disturbed anymore.

I believed that this young fellow was the one who pulled out the beautiful dahlias.

It was not my own making!

41

JESUS CHRIST APPEARED BEFORE ME!

I would like to relate again this most extraordinary and unbelievable experience which I had regarding the appearance of Jesus Christ.

"On the eve of my 48th birthday, in September 1985, a spectacular and marvellous event happened. For a long time, I have asked myself whether I should include this incident in this book. A lot of people might think that I could have hallucinated. There is no figment of doubt that this was coincidental or delusional. I leave this matter to the reader to believe or not. What occurred and what I saw vividly with my own eyes was undeniably true.

On that day, I had my cup of coffee at the back of my clinic. (Clinic is called surgery here in Australia.) At 11 o'clock in the morning while standing at the back porch, I looked at the beautiful cloud formations in the western sky. They appeared in different sizes, quite apart from each other. Some were thick, others bulky and dense. They moved gently and were almost unnoticeable across the blue sky.

This reminded me of an incident that took place when I was about nine years old. Many times I would lay down for a long time on the ground or on a piece of timber late in the afternoon and gaze at the sky and the silvery clouds. My eyes followed them for long periods, perhaps for 20 minutes or longer. I was charmed by the unique configurations they formed one minute and appearing in different shapes at the next.

I was also reminded of a couple of experiences, first in Mount Talinis, Negros Oriental, when a huge tunnel or hole formed inside a big cloud, enabling Jim Paton (an exchange student from Ohio) and myself to see the lowlands, and second, in Mount Canlaon when clouds danced before me.

That morning, as I was watching the clouds at the back of my clinic, an idea came to my mind. Why not try psychokinesis? I relaxed and leaned on the brick wall. Focusing my vision on one particular dense cumulus cloud, I did mind projection -- telling a particular cloud to disperse. Disperse! Disperse! Disperse! After two or three minutes that cloud vanished! The other clouds nearby remained intact. I tried another much bigger white bulbous cloud. This disappeared too. That thrilled me! A surge of adrenalin made my heart beat rapidly for a minute. I wondered if this was really psychokinesis. Or was it chance? Clouds usually form and disappear but they took much longer to disperse than when I told them to disappear.

The following day, I practiced dispersing clouds and let the video camera roll and then checking if they disappeared. By not doing psychokinesis on a particular cloud, smaller formations dispersed by themselves but then new ones would form somewhere nearby. The much denser and larger cumulus clouds did not vanish by themselves but stayed on until they could no longer be seen in the horizon.

At one moment, a huge nimbus cloud was looming in the sky. A dark grey rain-bearing cloud, all bunched together, was occupying almost a quarter of the open sky. I fixed my focus for a few minutes. I told this cloud, in my mind, to disperse. It did not disperse, but a large hole formed inside the cloud. The large tunnel disappeared later in two or three minutes. Strange, that I could do psychokinesis. Did I? Was there some mystical force behind what I was doing? I was skeptical. I got puzzled. Is this really psychokinesis? How many people can do this?

I practised on a few clouds in the stratosphere where the air current was very slow. It took a longer time to disperse them but they also vanished. All this I kept to myself. Every time I got a break and when darker cumulus cloud formations emerged, I practiced psychokinesis. I found this relaxing, especially the muscles behind the back of my neck.

On the eve of my 48th birthday, I had my coffee break at about 11 o'clock in the morning. I went to the back porch. As I sipped my cup of hot coffee slowly, I thought to myself that I could not possibly disperse any cloud this time as clouds were moving very fast. It was windy. The clouds came from the east, faster than usual. The weather during springtime can be unpredictable as we all know in Australia.

At that hour, Typhoon Gloria was lashing in Florida., USA. I conversed with myself, "Why not?" If this power can be applied with the help of the Supernatural Force, I might be able to slow down a hurricane." What a crazy thought!

As I concentrated on the large columns of dense bulbous clouds rushing from the east, I tried to disperse one cloud formation but the clouds moved fast, splitting by themselves, and rushing westward with the strong winds. I could not pick one for practice.

At a distance, there was a solid white cloud, silvery, that moved slowly. Why would this cloud move sluggishly compared with the rest? I concentrated on this unusual cloud for two to three minutes. Nothing happened.

When it was directly above my head, that cloud stopped! This was strange! A figure appeared on the cloud, or rather, the cloud formed itself into a figure with a head, followed by the neck, the upper part of the body, and shoulders. Then around the head sharp spokes appeared pointing outwards. This was a very strange phenomenon that was taking place! I could not blink! The whole picture that appeared resembled the Statue of Liberty! That stunned me! I could not move; I fixed my eyes on the figure-formation above me. That portrait stayed for a few seconds. Afterwards, the sharp pointed rays around the head folded and entwined upon each other, forming a thorny crown.

THE HEAD, FACE, NECK, AND UPPER HALF OF THE BODY OF JESUS CHRIST APPEARED BEFORE ME!

He had a sad face as if He was still hanging on the Cross looking down at me! It looked as if blood was dripping from His forehead!

I was absolutely stunned for a brief moment! Subsequently, the whole solid cloud with His face, neck, upper body and shoulders moved slowly towards the west, His face still looking down at me. I followed Him with my eyes. It must have been 30 seconds or more but His face did not dissipate. And then I remembered I had a video camera in my office. I jumped to get it, hoping I could take a shot of His face.

When I returned the solid cloud had scattered into many smaller silvery clouds. Why did it not stay as a solid cloud? I went inside the house, amazed at the spectacle.

My mother, sewing in the kitchen, saw me rushing in and rushing out. She asked, "What's happening?"

"I saw Jesus Christ in the cloud and I wanted to take a picture of Him," I answered, and added, "But the cloud has dissipated!"

She looked at me intently without saying anything. She probably thought I was crazy!

To me, the psychokinetic exercise I did a few days before this episode was a prelude to what was to be displayed in that precise hour. It never occurred to me that it would lead to this exposure.

I am an expressed believer in reincarnation. Why was this revelation shown to me? Did others see the unique cloud formation above the city of Blacktown, New South Wales? I guess nobody would be aware of the spiritual meaning of clouds that pass overhead every hour of the day.

Nonetheless, I believe in a Universal God and I claim no particular creed. I believe in the universality and oneness of God for all humankind. I have respect for all other religions of the world, great or otherwise. The important consideration is how one practices the tenets of one's religious affiliation. After all, it has been the religious dogmas that have played major roles in molding the systems of morality of millions of people in all continents.

In the early existence of man, God saw the future and anticipated that there would be many religious orders. Messages were written by messengers of God. One of these is exemplified in the Book of Micah in the Old Testament, Chapter 6, verse 8 which states... "What doth the Lord require of thee, but to do justly, to love mercy, and to walk humbly with thy God." Many will interpret this in different ways. "To walk humbly with Thy God" will not connote that there is a god for every religion.

If one, for instance, does not open one's mind to the concepts and precepts of other faiths, a degree of fanaticism may directly influence one's thoughts. One may condemn the beliefs of others as a "snare of the devil."

Can one really show mercy to all and claim one walks humbly with his god but in one's heart there abide intolerance and greed? This is hypocrisy in its terrible form. Such outlook could be directed by one's faith and one's own belief in God, but in reality we are all under one God. Would this be a better world if we had one government and one religion?

It is easier to follow a religious dogma or be indoctrinated into it than to accept a new one. I have become so open-minded that I cannot accept a particular religious teaching as the one and true teaching.

We may worship different gods, but we all know there is only one God. Whether one is a Japanese Shintoist, an Australian Anglican, a Vietnamese Buddhist, an African Atheist, a Chinese Catholic, or an American Protestant, or whatever nationality or race one may belong to--we are all under one Creator.

Every human being has a soul which has a long thorny road to traverse towards perfection. Except for open-minded individuals, I doubt if reincarnation would find acceptance among religious groups.

I am happy and contented, for 'Fear of the Lord is the beginning of wisdom.'

The appearance of Jesus Christ in the cloud was the most revealing encounter I had experienced in my life.

Does God have a design for me? Why did Jesus appear to me?

I am waiting for the answer. It has been 28 years since Jesus appeared to me.

42

ELIJAH, THE HOLY GHOST!

On October 10, 1985, I was told by Mrs. Pam P. (a very good clairvoyant) in one of her "readings" *that I should open my Bible the following morningy and, without looking, point my right index finger to a verse.*

'When you get up tomorrow morning, open the Bible, with eyes closed, flip it once, and point your finger blindly to a verse, and *a message will be given to you,*' said the reading.

The next day, I opened the Bible and placed my right forefinger blindly on a verse on a page. The verse was John 16:13, which read,

'Howbeit, when he, the Spirit of truth, is come, he will guide you into all truth: for he shall not speak of himself: but whatsoever he shall hear, that he shall speak: and he will show you things to come.'

What are the chances of my reopening the Bible and pointing my finger blindly to this particular verse? One in a million or more! But if one has guidance from an unknown force it will exactly point to the exact verse. Is it by chance?

Many Pentecostals and some other religious groups believe that the Holy Spirit will dwell in you (believers) and you are healed of your ailment and you will speak in tongues. I have attended a few meetings among Pentecostals in the past – but the words that came out of their mouths could not be understood. They were just mumblings.

The newer version (The Gideon's International) reads:

'When the Spirit of Truth comes, however, He will guide you into all truth.'

I called Mrs. Pam P. on the telephone that very minute I read John 16:13. She said, **'The message is in the second half of the verse.'** The amazing thing is that Mrs. Pam P did not know much of the Bible.

What was the second part of the verse? **'For he will not speak on his own account but whatever he** *hears* (the person called by the Holy Ghost) **and he will make known to you what is to take place.'**

A prophecy is written in the last chapter of the Old Testament. Malachai 4:5 says, **'Behold, I will send you Elijah, the prophet before the coming of the great dreadful day of the Lord.'**

This verse tells of God sending Elijah, but not in his person as when he appeared from Gilead 3,000 years ago, but through a person he will possess.

The interpretation that the Holy Ghost or the Comforter was sent by God right after the death of Jesus Christ has been accepted by many Christian denominations. The doctrine of the Holy Trinity was based upon this.

The Bible says there is one God. Jesus (in the flesh) manifested heavenly wonders as the Son of God.

There is one Holy Ghost. The Holy Ghost is Elijah who will be sent again in the early part of the 21st century to fulfil the long-standing prophecies. He cannot be the Holy Ghost who can be everywhere. When Elijah comes, will he be in many places? No. Just in one place. He will probably use television or the mass media to announce himself.

How will Elijah come? It will not be the same appearance as he appeared 3,000 years ago when he came out of the wilderness. With God's plan, Elijah will have to use a servant destined to carry out the prophecies.

The doctrine of the Trinity has been a divisive issue throughout the entire history of the Christian church. While the core aspects of the Trinity are clearly presented in God's Word, some of the side issues are not as explicitly clear. The Father is God, the Son is God, and the Holy Spirit is God—but there is only one God.

Beyond that, the issues are, to a certain extent, debatable and non-essential. Rather than attempting to fully define the Trinity with our finite human minds, we would be better off focusing on the fact of God's greatness and His infinitely higher nature of love and light.

Romans 11:33-34 states: 'Oh, how can you measure the depth of the riches of the wisdom and knowledge of the Creator? How unsearchable his judgments, and his paths beyond tracing out! Who has known the mind of the Lord? Or who has been the Counselor?'

Was the Bible really the altered of extraterrestrials by controlling the minds of the writer?

Recent disclosures have been made by some people who had contact with aliens, who took them to their planets, and met with the prophets, even Jesus Christ. It is for us to accept and believe that there is nothing evil but good in these encounters.

Did Jesus see Satan when he was tempted in the mount? He is mentioned in the New Testament as saying, 'Get away from me, Satan!'

43

'I HAVE CALLED THEE!'

At 4:44 a.m., on the 29th of July 1986 (in Blacktown, New South Wales where I practiced family medicine since 1979) I was awakened by a sudden unusual sound in the room. I could not tell what woke me up. I looked at the radio clock above my headboard: it was exactly 4:44 in the morning. That was my first time to see this number. A second later, I felt something on the right palm of my hand. I switched on the light (lampshade) by my side and I saw a small piece of paper. This measured exactly 1.25 x 1 inch with the beautiful print, **"I have called Thee."** Underneath this line was Is. 43:1.

Since that time the number 444 kept coming to me. Whenever I glanced at my watch or the office clock the number would be 4:44 in the morning or in the afternoon at least once every week. Many years passed, and I still kept getting the reminder – No. 444.

After 11 years the number 444 stopped coming to me. It has been replaced by the number 222, which comes very often these days I know now what the numbers 444 and 222 meant. I will tell you the meaning of this in due time.

'I Have Called Thee!'

This message is found in Isaiah 43:1. For a long time I did not know of the prophecy of the coming of Elijah.

> Prophet Elijah told the Israelites that an offspring from the East, a soul related, not a physical descendant, will come from the east.
>
> He tells us in Isaiah 46:11, '**From the east** I summon a bird of prey; from a far-off land, **a man to fulfill my purpose**. What I have said, that will I bring about; what I have planned, that will I do.' Even the birds are

somehow part of His preordained plan. **Furthermore, there are times when He chooses to let us know His plans** (Isaiah 46:10)

This is in collaboration with The Prophesy made by Edgar Cayce about **Xerxes** who will appear in the latter days. In the previous life (incarnation), Xerxes was King David of Israel. Of course one cannot believe this statement if one does not believe in reincarnation.

The time is ripe and the change to a New Social Order will slowly take place. This will be after the AWFUL HOUR. How will the public be convinced without getting into a panic? A portion of the video of Inelia Benz showed that she was speaking in Spanish but a listener told her that she spoke in Portuguese.

When the time comes for me to complete my mission, my guides will use me as promised, that when I hear the voice dictate to me, the listener will hear it in their own tongue. This will be seen on television and heard over the radio. It sounds crazy. I have asked some friends if I showed signs of craziness and they said no.

This is the process that will convince the non-believers that truly we are created by good aliens who want to save the planet. If they were malevolent, they would have exterminated us with their advanced technology a long time ago. Where do the good aliens or benevolent come from? From the Source.

III

THE FIRST MESSAGE ON MY ARM

P ast Revelation--" I HAVE CALLED THEE" JULY 29, 1986 at 4:44 A.M.
August, 1986 to February 2023 ------------------------------- 444 months
This is based on the communication I received in July 29, 1986, on an small old stamp.

The predictions made by some contactees, including the Mayan predictions foretold this to happen in 2012... but was post poned. Who deferred this?

"Search and you will find."

Some prophecies happen in the exact hour, in country and individuals. Some prophecies are known to be flexible and some don't happen at all. Are these influencd by the good vibrations of the collective human mind?

THE RECENT PERSONAL REVELATION
THE FIRST MESSAGE ON MY RIGHT FOREARM

An elevated mark on my right volar aspect of my right forearm appeared on late afternoon of the 8th of February 2014. (Note: I don't have a medical condition known as Dermatographia.) *This lasted more than 4 hours. I took pictures of this.*

The mark *showed in Roman Numeral -- 'XXII. (Meaning year 2022)*

Is this the beginning of the levelling of mankind or The AWFUL HOUR? A Geologic Cataclysm?

Will this occur in the YEAR 2022! Can this major prophecy be averted! It is humanity's card on the table. Learn the vibratory lessons recommented by Inelia Benz and her group. Inelia Benz has no reord of previous reincarnation. She was sent directly from above. Inelia will be leaving us soon. She is going back to the Source in April 2017.

IV

THE SECOND MESSAGE WRITTEN ON MY RIGHT FOREARM

A year later, February 2015, a second message appeared on my right forearm. It also appeared in Roman Numeral: XX1. The global cataclysm will then occur on 2021. Six years from this writing.

Man is not changing at all. His attitude towards his neighbour has gotten worse. Jesus said 2000 years ago: "This generation is wicked and adulterous." God may shorten the time but no one knows.

CONCLUSION

Has this book changed your life after reading this? You do have a commitment to your soul but have not realized this. The choice is yours!

My beloved brothers and sisters in Him, it is my wish that you make a positive choice. The END of the cycles is almost here. What is five years compared to 12,000 years? Our flesh returns to dust but the soul lives on forever.

You might not believe this because it has not happened yet. if you act later and admit that I was right that I was a messenger of God, it might be too late! Would you act or not act as many have done in the past. They did not believe the prophets during their time.

Let us be reminded of one of the messages of Jesus, one of the Ascended Masters, when he spoke in Matthew 13:48.. "The angels of the Lord will come forth and separate the wicked from the just."

The way the angels will treat you is your own making. Then you will have to reincarnate again and again until the mission of the soul is fullfilled or if the your karma is very heavy you will be brought to a distant plant and incarnate with the lower arimals of that planet for millions of years.

When you attend celebrations with a big crowd gatherings by the thousands in areas of sports, all thoughts, actions and all undertakings are listed down? But sad to say, none of them is ever conscious of God's ways.

"In all thy ways, acknowledge Him and He will direct thy paths". Proverbs 3:2.

Have you? Establish that conscionsness that a dazzling partlicle of God is in every human heart ready to respond to your call. When you decide to make the call stick to it until the end of your earthly life and not going back a countless times through the process of reincarnation.

THE END

Printed in the United States
By Bookmasters